UNLEASH the
INNER
HEALING
POWER
of FOODS

By the Editors of FC&A Medical Publishing®

Publisher's Note

The editors of FC&A have taken careful measures to ensure the accuracy and usefulness of the information in this book. While every attempt has been made to assure accuracy, errors may occur. We advise readers to carefully review and understand the ideas and tips presented and to seek the advice of a qualified professional before attempting to use them. The publisher and editors disclaim all liability (including any injuries, damages or losses) resulting from the use of the information in this book.

The health information in this book is for information only and is not intended to be a medical guide for self-treatment. It does not constitute medical advice and should not be construed as such or used in place of your doctor's medical advice.

" **Now I exhort you, brethren, by the name of our Lord Jesus Christ, that you all agree and that there be no divisions among you, but that you be made complete in the same mind and in the same judgement.**"

1 Corinthians 1:10

FC&A
103 Clover Green
Peachtree City, GA 30269
www.fca.com

Produced by the staff of FC&A

First printing April 2003

ISBN 1-890957-77-1

Table of Contents

CHAPTER 1 *Allergies*

What are allergies? You are considered allergic if your immune system overreacts to a normally harmless substance, called an allergen. Common allergens are mold, pollen, dust, and pet dander. Foods, like peanuts, can also trigger an allergic reaction.

Who gets them? Allergies affect more than 20 percent of Americans. They often run in families, but you can also get them from repeated exposure to common allergens. For instance, health care workers might develop a latex allergy from wearing latex gloves every day.

What are common symptoms? Skin rash, scratchy or swollen throat, watery eyes, stuffy or runny nose, sneezing, sinus headaches, difficulty breathing, stomach upset, vomiting, diarrhea, or bloating.

Delicious ways to dodge food allergies

You may not want to kiss and tell, but one woman couldn't help it after kissing her husband. She is allergic to peanuts. He just ate a nutty candy bar. The result – itching and swelling serious enough to require medication.

According to the National Institute of Allergy and Infectious Diseases, one in three people in America think they have food allergies. But in reality, only about 1 percent of the population has an authentic immune system reaction.

The hallmark of a true allergy is its speed. From hives to wheezing to anaphylactic shock – a sudden, often fatal drop in blood pressure – you'll experience allergic symptoms within the hour.

You can blame over 90 percent of all food allergies on just eight edibles – peanuts, tree nuts (walnuts, cashews, pecans, etc.), milk, eggs, wheat, fish, shellfish, and soy. There is no cure, so prevention is truly your best medicine. Here are some tips to help you avoid an unhealthy encounter.

If you've been allergic to peanuts since childhood, ask your doctor about a peanut allergy test. You might be among the 20 percent who have outgrown this nutty reaction.

Tree nuts and peanuts. Nuts are hidden in some unusual places – barbecue sauce, crackers, ethnic foods, and baked goods, for example. If you're allergic, even casual contact with a nut-laden food or a food prepared alongside nuts can cause anaphylaxis.

Carefully examine all food labels, and not just the ingredients list, for the word nut or peanut. Alert your waiter at every restaurant to the seriousness of your allergy. He can help make sure your meal isn't cross-contaminated. And be especially wary of restaurant desserts and home-baked goodies.

To add a satisfying crunch to dishes without touching a nut, mix in rice crispies, candy pieces, crunchy fresh vegetables, or dried fruit.

Milk. Dairy doesn't just come in cartons. Check labels because you may find these milk by-products in lots of foods: casein, sodium caseinate, lactose, and whey. Also check that the meat slicer in your deli is not also used for cheese.

Lactose intolerance, a digestive sensitivity to dairy, has made substitutes like rice and soy milks readily available. In recipes, you can also replace milk with an equal amount of water or fruit juice.

Eggs. Like milk, you must look for ingredients derived from eggs. Food labels may list them as albumin, globulin, or ovomucin. Be especially careful with foamy drinks and commercially prepared pasta – many contain eggs.

The Food Allergy and Anaphylaxis Network says if a home recipe calls for eggs, try mixing up one of these. Each mixture can be substituted for one egg.

- 1 teaspoon baking powder plus 1 tablespoon any liquid, and 1 tablespoon vinegar

- 1 teaspoon yeast dissolved in 1/4 cup warm water

- 1 1/2 tablespoons water plus 1 1/2 tablespoons vegetable oil, and 1 teaspoon baking powder

- 1 packet gelatin mixed with 2 tablespoons warm water

Wheat. Products that contain hidden wheat include bulgur, couscous, beer, white vinegar, hot dogs, ice cream, and many pastas. In addition, wheat flour is used as a thickener in everything from casseroles to soups. Check labels carefully for any mention of gluten, semolina, food starch, bran, HVP, or MSG. These usually refer to wheat products.

A wheat allergy is different from celiac disease (celiac sprue). Suffering from celiac sprue means avoiding gluten-containing foods all your life.

At home, put tofu or cooked rice through a blender and use to thicken soups. Corn starch will also thicken sauces. You can replace a cup of wheat flour in home recipes with any one of the following:

- 7/8 cup rice flour

- 5/8 cup potato starch flour

- 1 cup soy flour plus 1/4 cup potato starch flour

- 1 cup corn flour

Try picking up a loaf of rye, oat, or barley bread instead of wheat bread. But still check the ingredients list just to be safe.

Fish and shellfish. Flying fish in the Atlantic ocean use their wing-like fins to glide over the surface of the water. But they're not the only seafood that's going airborne. Fish particles are light enough to float in the air, making open-air markets and fish stalls dangerous places if you're allergic to seafood. It's possible to breathe in these fish particles and suffer a reaction.

Since you risk anaphylactic shock with a fish allergy, make sure you also check labels on condiments for anchovies or other fish products.

Omega-3 oils are crucial fatty acids that help your body fight inflammation. If you're avoiding fish – the richest food source of omega-3 oil – eat plenty of plant sources instead, like flaxseed or dark green leafy vegetables.

Soy. Also known as miso, tofu, tempeh, or vegetable protein, soy has been a mainstay of Asian diets for centuries. Because it doesn't have its own distinct flavor, soy is used in many packaged products – even chocolate. Read the labeling fine print carefully, since it's very easy to miss.

Because of the nature of food allergies, you may want to cook most of your meals from scratch. This gives you control over all ingredients. There are plenty of allergy cookbooks that can help you avoid anything from milk to mushrooms. Look for them at your local library or bookstore.

Rotate foods to fix allergies

Some allergy-prone individuals swear by the rotation diet, an eating plan that groups foods and limits how often you eat them. In this way, experts believe you can:

- prevent new food allergies

- pinpoint specific foods you are allergic to

- continue eating foods you have only mild reactions to

In her book, *5 Years Without Food: The Food Allergy Survival Guide*, Nicholette Dumke explains how avoiding problem foods doesn't stop food sensitivi-ties. Instead, many people develop reactions to the foods they continue eating. "Any

Watch out for these subtle symptoms of food sensitivity: fatigue, migraines, obesity, even arthritis.

food," she says, "if eaten repetitively, can cause food aller-gies in allergy-prone individuals."

The solution – rotate foods so your body doesn't become sensi-tive to any one food. Here are the nuts and bolts of a typical rotation diet.

- Eliminate all the foods you are sensitive to. Keep a food diary and ask your doctor about allergy tests to find out what these may be.

- Learn how to group the remaining foods into families. You'll need a reference list from your doctor or one like that found in Dumke's book. "Foods are rotated according to their bio-logical classification in food families," Dumke explains, "because foods in the same family have similar antigens."

- Depending on how severe your food allergies are, your doc-tor may vary how strict your rotation should be. Most rota-tion cycles are four to five days long.

- Once your symptoms are gone and you're feeling well, you can gradually add the problem foods back into your diet. "Eat your problem foods in moderate amounts and on a strictly rotated basis," says Dumke. You'll need to cut back the minute symptoms return.

While on this diet, it's important to follow good nutrition guidelines. Since there are many food families, you can still put together a healthy plate – a mix of produce, grains, and protein. "A highly varied diet is the most healthy kind of diet for everyone to eat," says Dumke. Think of it as a wonderful opportunity to add foods to your menu that you've never tried before.

- Protein isn't exclusive to chicken, beef, or pork. Venison, buffalo, rabbit, goat, ostrich, lamb, wild boar, goose, or quail are all excellent alternatives. Perch, catfish, roughy, halibut, and sardines expand your seafood vocabulary, and don't forget wild bird and ostrich eggs, goat and sheep cheeses, and beans.

- Don't rely on wheat. Try some of these less appreciated grains – amaranth, buckwheat, cassava, kamut, millet, oats, quinoa, spelt, teff, and wild rice.

- Go for the forgotten vegetables like artichokes, leeks, sorrel, chard, endives, and parsnips. Add chickpeas, beans, and various nuts and seeds for extra crunch.

- Finally, add interest to your fruit bowl with figs, muscadines, pumellos, persimmons, star fruit, or mangoes.

If you want to try this diet, talk to your doctor or nutritionist. They can give you more details and supervise your diet so you don't leave any important nutrients out. "Once you get used to your rotation diet," says Dumke, "it will become easier to use and your health will be improved by using it."

Get sneeze-free with a smarter diet

What do green tea, buckwheat, kiwis, and fish have in common? These four foods are all natural antihistamines that can help open your stuffy nose without drugs. Here's how.

To stop an allergic reaction in its tracks, you need to block histamine release. Dr. Gailen D. Marshall Jr., Director of the Division of Allergy and Clinical Immunology at the University of Texas Houston Medical School, describes what happens in your body when your immune system encounters a specific kind of pollen.

"Your immune system is designed to protect 'me' (your body). It will go around and look at substances it encounters in the body and ask, 'Is that me? Is that not me?' After deciding 'It's not me,' the next question is 'Is it capable of creating disease?' For people that are not allergic to a pollen, the normal answer is 'no.' But in an allergic person, the immune system gets confused and thinks it's a bad thing."

This triggers an allergic reaction and your immune system releases histamine, which can cause a host of symptoms including itching, sneezing, coughing, and wheezing.

That's when antihistamines provide welcome relief.

Brew a pot of green tea. A powerful antioxidant in green tea appears to interfere with your body's allergy response before it even starts. It not only blocks the production of histamines, but also shuts down the receptors that tell your body to react to allergens.

Green tea is generally thought safe, but experts want more human studies before deciding how much and which green teas work best.

Flip for buckwheat flapjacks. Quercetin is a natural chemical in certain plants that just may prevent your next sneezing attack. It acts like a commercial antihistamine, regulating the membranes in your body that release histamine. Buckwheat is a good source but you can also find quercetin in apples, onions, and citrus fruits. It's available as a supplement, too, but talk to your doctor before taking it.

> **To clear your sinuses, dissolve a half teaspoon of salt in a cup of warm water. With a bulb syringe, flush your nose with the mixture.**

Cash in on kiwis. This fuzzy fruit is loaded with vitamin C which may keep your white blood cells from releasing histamine, and disarm histamine once it is released. In fact, if you don't get enough vitamin C, your histamine levels go up, along with your chances of suffering from allergies.

"There is evidence," Marshall says, "that vitamin C has been a long-term remedy for certain kinds of allergies." But, he points out, you must take it regularly and not just as allergies attack. Research shows you can safely take one gram of vitamin C a day from supplements and natural sources.

Other foods that boost your C power are red and green peppers, broccoli, cabbage, citrus fruits, berries, and guavas.

Feast on fish. Allergy sufferers want a healthy dose of niacin, a member of the B vitamin family. It prevents your cells from releasing histamine. Fish, lean meats, and beans are all good sources.

To keep your immune system stable, it's important to get enough omega-3 fatty acids. Fish like tuna and salmon are rich in omega-3 and will help balance out the inflammation-prone omega-6 fatty acids in your body.

Marshall says taking an omega-3 supplement won't hurt, but make sure you mention it to your doctor in case it interferes with your other medications.

If changes in your diet have no effect on your allergies, Marshall enthusiastically recommends the newest development in allergy treatment – immunotherapy. This allergy vaccine program can help people allergic to pollen, dust, and bug bites.

"When it works, allergen immunotherapy re-educates the immune system to stop recognizing pollen, for instance, as harmful," Marshall says. This could mean permanent relief for your allergy symptoms. Because there are so many different combinations of allergies, ask your doctor if these shots are for you.

Healthy habits

Your best line of defense against allergy attacks is to avoid allergens and keep your body in shape. Here are some tips to help you do both.

- Check pollen counts in the newspaper or on your local weather channel. If they are high, stay inside.
- Take a shower as soon as you come in from outdoors to wash pollen from your hair and skin.
- Exercise indoors.
- Keep the humidity in your home below 50 percent to discourage mold.
- Wash your bedding once a week in hot water. This will kill dust mites.
- Throw your clothes in the dryer instead of hanging them outside where they can pick up a variety of pollen and mold spores.
- Switch to feather pillows. Synthetic pillows are proven to contain more allergens.
- Dry steam clean your carpets and upholstered furniture regularly to get rid of mites.
- Cut down on dust inside by keeping doors and windows closed and knickknacks to a minimum.

CHAPTER 2 *Alzheimer's disease*

What is Alzheimer's disease? It's a common form of dementia, or severe loss of mental ability, that interferes with everyday life. Alzheimer's affects the part of the brain that controls memory, speech, and thinking. It develops gradually and is irreversible.

Who gets it? One in 10 people over age 65 and nearly half over age 85 develop Alzheimer's. Blacks, smokers, people with a history of high blood pressure, those who have had a head injury, especially a serious one, are at greatest risk.

What are the symptoms? Gradual loss of memory, confusion, difficulty in making decisions, inability to learn new information, language difficulties, anxiety, depression, and personality changes.

Why you need to eat fish and nuts

It may sound nutty, even a little bit fishy, but the foods you eat really do affect your brain. Walnuts, almonds, and other nuts, as well as cold water fish, like salmon, tuna, and mackerel, give you lots of omega-3 fatty acids. This form of unsaturated fat helps improve your brain's performance and your memory.

One study found that older people who eat fish at least once a week are less likely to develop Alzheimer's disease (AD). The researchers also discovered the fish eaters were better educated than those who didn't eat fish, which may be partly responsible for the results. That's because using your brain seems to protect it. Nevertheless, fish improves blood flow to the brain and helps lower your risk of high cholesterol, heart disease, and stroke, making it a healthy addition to your diet.

You'll find both nuts and fish in the same group with meat, poultry, dry beans, and eggs on the USDA Food Pyramid. It's good to substitute these healthy fats for some of the saturated fat you eat in meat and cheese. But don't overdo the nuts. They have a lot of calories, and a high-calorie diet might increase your risk of Alzheimer's.

Almonds, ounce for ounce, provide nearly as much protein as red meat. They are cholesterol free, low in saturated fat, and high in vitamin E, calcium, and fiber.

Fish, on the other hand, provides omega-3 fatty acids with fewer calories per ounce, so it's safe to help yourself to more generous servings. You may be tempted to bake your fish in a crust of almonds for a delicious combination of the two. But for the most nutrition, it's better to eat nuts raw.

'Vaccinate' your brain with vitamins

A simple vaccination may someday remove your fears about getting Alzheimer's disease. But you don't have to wait for years of development and testing to start protecting yourself against this memory-robbing disease. You can start creating your own "vaccination" right now with a diet that's low in calories and fat and high in these vitamins.

Vitamin E. You may more than double your protection against Alzheimer's just by increasing this one vitamin in your diet. "The more vitamin E that people consumed in their diets from foods, the lower their risk of developing AD," says researcher Martha Clare Morris. She and fellow scientists at Chicago's Rush Institute for Healthy Aging and Rush-Presbyterian-St. Luke's Medical Center found that people who got the most vitamin E from foods lowered their risk an astounding 67 percent when compared with those in the study who got the lowest amounts.

"The results of this study provide the most direct evidence to date of a link between dietary vitamin E and AD," said Morris. Supplements, however, didn't provide the same benefit.

The experts think it's the antioxidant quality of vitamin E-rich foods, like cantaloupe, green leafy vegetables, seeds and nuts, olive oil, and whole grain breads and cereals, that made the difference for people in the study. These foods help reduce free radical damage that scientists link to both Alzheimer's and heart disease. Unfortunately, the beneficial results of this study didn't hold true for people with a genetic link to Alzheimer's.

But vitamin E is just the start in creating your AD "vaccine." A variety of other nutrients will also help to hold Alzheimer's at bay.

Vitamin C. A tossed salad – with tomatoes, red and yellow peppers, carrots, and dark greens – is an easy way to work brain-saving nutrition into your diet. You'll not only get lots of vitamin C, you'll be loading up on other antioxidants, like vitamin E, beta carotene, and a variety of flavonoids.

Apples, oranges, bananas, strawberries, and blueberries are some of the fruits and berries also loaded with antioxidants. Enjoy them on cereal, in salads, or by themselves as snacks. When possible, eat the skins of fruits and vegetables, too. The extra fiber adds even more protection for your brain by lowering cholesterol and blood pressure, both linked to Alzheimer's.

> **Create a salad for your brain with avocado slices and mandarin oranges on a bed of greens. Top it off with a few slivered almonds and a low-fat vinaigrette dressing.**

B vitamins. Eat a variety of whole grains – brown rice, whole wheat bread, and oat bran cereal are good choices. Add nuts, beans, leafy green vegetables, and salmon or other fish. What you'll get are lots of B vitamins for your brain, including B12 and folate, two of the most important ones.

"In our study, we found that low levels of either of these two vitamins were related to an increased Alzheimer's disease risk," says Hui-Xin Wang, a researcher with the Swedish Kungsholmen Project. His study monitored the levels of these vital nutrients in 370 healthy people age 75 and older for three years.

A regular 12-ounce cafe latte supplies 400 mg of calcium. You can get even more calcium, and less fat and calories, by using low-fat or fat-free milk.

People with low amounts of B12 and folate had higher homocysteine levels. This is particularly important because one study found that people with high levels of homocysteine were at an almost three times greater risk for Alzheimer's disease than those with low levels.

Other researchers have found B6 also helps lower homocysteine. Still others discovered that B12 and thiamin, another B vitamin found in whole grains, nuts, and beans, help carry messages quickly to and from your brain.

Calcium. This is the first major mineral your mother provided you as an infant, and it may be the key to staying sharp throughout your life. It helps your brain and nerve cells work together and helps protect you from bone loss, too. This makes calcium a strong addition to your AD vaccine.

You probably think first of milk when you think of calcium. And low-fat dairy products are a good source, but don't forget these other ways to get more calcium.

- Start the day with calcium-fortified oatmeal and a glass of calcium-fortified orange juice.

- Enjoy some sardines or salmon canned with bones.

- Go for greens – broccoli, spinach, Swiss chard, kale, beet greens, or turnip greens.

Enhance brainpower with ancient herb

Increase blood flow to your brain, improve your thinking, and slow down the progression of Alzheimer's disease with an ancient remedy – ginkgo.

For over 5,000 years, the Chinese have been using the leaf of the ginkgo biloba tree to increase circulation and boost memory. So why shouldn't it work today?

Modern scientists studying the effects of ginkgo extract on the progression of Alzheimer's, however, seemed to get mixed results. But recently researchers took a second look at 33 studies and threw out those that were not reliable. Based on the well-done studies, both the safety and effectiveness of the extract look promising.

"The medicinal effects of ginkgo," says researcher Dr. James Warner of Imperial College London, "are believed to be gained by causing blood vessels to dilate, improving blood flow to the brain, and through thinning the blood and making it less likely to clot."

And that's not all. "Ginkgo," Warner continues, "probably also has some antioxidant effects, protecting nerve cells against biological 'rusting.'" This explains why ginkgo not only helps fend off Alzheimer's, but also helps you battle heart disease, stroke, and other diseases.

> **If you help care for someone who has Alzheimer's disease, steer him away from alcohol. Not only does it destroy brain cells, it can interfere with Alzheimer's medications.**

Look in health food stores for ginkgo biloba leaf extract that contains 24 percent to 26 percent flavonoid glycosides and 5 percent to 7 percent terpene lactones. The recommended dose is 120 milligrams (mg) broken down into 40 mg to 60 mg doses throughout the day.

Don't take ginkgo along with aspirin, warfarin, or any other blood-thinning medication. And be patient. It could take four to six weeks for the full effect to kick in.

Remarkable way to outsmart Alzheimer's

Protection from Alzheimer's disease may come from a surprising source – cholesterol-lowering drugs. According to a study at the Boston University School of Medicine, commonly prescribed drugs called statins could lower your risk of developing Alzheimer's.

"This study confirms and extends previous reports and is the largest study on this topic in the U.S.," says lead researcher Dr. Robert C. Green. Following 2,581 people for six years, researchers found that people taking statins had an amazing 79 percent reduction in risk of AD.

The study was the first, Green notes, to include a large number of blacks – a group especially at risk for AD. The good news is statins protect blacks and whites equally.

The results are also the same for those who carry the gene associated with AD and those who don't. One theory suggests statins might prevent Alzheimer's by reducing inflammation in the brain.

Some studies show a connection between Alzheimer's and high cholesterol, but in this study, other cholesterol-lowering drugs didn't reduce AD risk.

Health professionals don't recommend taking statins just as protection against AD. And if you do take statins for high cholesterol, they urge you to report any numbness, tingling, or pain in your hands and feet to your doctor. These are symptoms of nerve damage, which can be a side effect of statins.

Healthy habits

You can lower your Alzheimer's risk with an active, challenging lifestyle.

- Look for new interests that challenge and stretch your gray matter.
- Get together frequently with old friends and new.
- Talk with your doctor about taking aspirin every day.
- Exercise regularly.
- Watch your step, use your seat belt, wear a helmet if you bike or rollerblade, and take tai chi classes for better balance to avoid head injuries.
- Keep cholesterol and blood pressure under control.
- Stop smoking.

CHAPTER 3

Asthma

What is asthma? It is a long-term lung disease caused by inflammation of the airways, which become sensitive and tighten up, making it difficult to breathe. Triggers for asthma attacks include allergens, other airborne irritants, respiratory infections, and exertion.

Who gets it? More than 25 million Americans – 2 million over age 65 – have had asthma during their lifetime. Asthma can occur at any age but often develops in childhood. It may go away and come back later in life.

What are the symptoms?

- wheezing and shortness of breath
- coughing, often accompanied by mucus
- chest tightness, especially in cold weather or exercise

An apple a day keeps asthma at bay

You can lower your chances of lung disease and even make your lungs work better just by eating a few vegetables and a little fruit each day – especially apples.

That's the conclusion of two British studies on chronic obstructive pulmonary disease (COPD), which can be caused by asthma, emphysema, and bronchitis.

A survey of heavy smokers revealed that eating just a portion of vegetables a day reduced the risk of COPD by almost half, and that one and a half portions of fruit, particularly apples, helped almost as much. Another study tested 2,633 adults and found that those who ate five apples a week could inhale and exhale a lot more air than those who didn't.

Three tomatoes a week produced the same result. Wheezing – a prime asthma symptom – was less common among those who ate apples, tomatoes, and bananas.

Breathing difficulty is the main symptom of asthma, so don't wait until it develops into the more serious pulmonary disease to start eating more fruits and vegetables.

Pick a juicy apple. Apples are a big plus in the fight against asthma. Apple skins contain lots of quercetin, a powerful antioxidant that helps keep asthma in check. And antioxidants battle the free radicals produced by your inflamed airways.

Scientists have proven that one small apple has as much antioxidant power as a 1,500-milligram vitamin C tablet. So eat apples – peelings and all – five times a week. Red onions, buckwheat, and citrus fruits are good sources of quercetin, too.

Set your sights on citrus fruits. Because it is the main antioxidant in the surface of the lung, vitamin C is a major player in the asthma game. Two surveys of the same people taken nine years apart showed that taking vitamin C over the long haul definitely helps maintain lung function.

Citrus fruits – oranges, grapefruit, lemons, and limes – are all near the top of the list of food sources for C. After that, it's "P" foods. Fill up on sweet peppers, peaches, papayas, and pineapple to get more vitamin C.

Look for the reddest tomatoes. Lycopene is a carotenoid that gives tomatoes their rich color. Since few foods have as much lycopene as tomatoes, that might be the reason a triple dose of them each week helps protect against asthma. You can also get lycopene from pink grapefruit and watermelon. Even better is guava, which compares to the tomato for lycopene and has more vitamin C than an orange. And about 30 dried apricots will provide the same amount of lycopene as one tomato.

Discover another kind of "apple." The mango is called the "apple of the tropics" and is also high in vitamin C. But it is loaded with other antioxidants, including vitamin E, which may help prevent asthma, especially in adults.

You may not be familiar with it, but people around the world eat more fresh mangoes than any other fruit. Give it a try, and you may soon count it among your favorites as well. Other foods with vitamin E are sweet potatoes and sunflower seeds.

Cut into a cantaloupe. Your body turns beta carotene into vitamin A, another powerful antioxidant that helps increase lung capacity. If you can't find mangoes – they have lots of beta carotene, too – try a cantaloupe. This juicy, delicious member of the gourd family has been pleasing people since 2,400 B.C. It gets its brilliant orange color from beta carotene, as do carrots and pumpkins.

Dine on a royal avocado. Compared to cantaloupes, the avocado is a relatively young tropical fruit. It only goes back to 291 B.C., when legend says a Mayan princess ate the first one. You can eat avocados for magnesium, which research has linked to higher lung capacity, especially when combined with vitamin C. This trace mineral acts as a bronchodilator to help open up your airways and make it easier to breathe. Magnesium also helps ease the muscle spasms of asthma attacks.

> Selenium, a trace mineral and an antioxidant, often works hand-in-hand with magnesium to quiet asthma. Get more of it by eating vegetables and grains grown in selenium-rich soil.

Soothe symptoms with bananas. This popular fruit, which helps cut down on wheezing, has another benefit for asthma sufferers. It helps soothe the indigestion that sometimes causes coughing. People with acid reflux – heartburn – often have asthma, too. Some scientists believe that stomach acid spilling into your airways can trigger asthma attacks. Whatever the reason, bananas will calm your cough and your indigestion while helping to eliminate your wheeze.

Healthy habits

You'll breathe easier if you asthma-proof one of the main gathering places in your home – the kitchen. Use these tips to get rid of common triggers and enjoy a more pleasant dining experience.

- Clean often to avoid grimy build-up that requires harsh chemical cleansers that trigger your asthma. Use hot soap and water to clean your counters, not irritating detergents.

- Don't wash with antibacterial soap. Research shows battling a few bacteria will actually stimulate your immune system and protect against allergies and related conditions like asthma.

- Wash dishes promptly. Dirty dishes in the sink encourage bacteria and invite cockroaches – a prime asthma trigger. Keep garbage containing food particles outside.

- Prevent mold by getting rid of moisture sources such as leaky pipes and wet carpet or ceiling tiles. Keep refrigerator drip pans clean and dry.

- Consider replacing your gas stove with an electric one. Nitrogen dioxide fumes from gas can create breathing problems. Exhaust fans take out smells and vapor but don't remove the fumes.

Break the food-asthma connection

Has eating a dried fig or apricot ever left you gasping for air? Did a glass of milk or wine start an uncontrollable cough? If so, you have experienced the connection between what you eat and how you breathe. By pinpointing the foods you're sensitive to, you can help avoid the inflammation that brings on your attacks.

Consider these foods first. Although almost any food can cause a reaction, the most common are eggs, milk, wheat, fish, citrus fruits, peanuts, and soy. These would be the first things to consider if you think a food sensitivity is causing your asthma attacks.

Other foods high on the list of allergens are shellfish, chocolate, and tree nuts. A recent Japanese study suggests that children who eat more fish may be more prone to asthma attacks.

Sometimes it's not the food itself, but something added to it, that causes your airways to close up. Sulfites are used to keep food looking fresh and give it a longer shelf life, but they are asthma triggers for some people. Products with sulfites include dried fruits, wine, beer, shrimp, bacon, cold cuts, and many packaged foods. Check package labels for possible triggers.

Even non-food items have been known to trigger asthma attacks. If you're asthmatic, stay away from royal jelly. This bee by-product has reportedly caused life-threatening asthma attacks. Aspirin and tartrazine, a dye found in some yellow food-coloring, can also be asthma triggers.

Keep a diet diary. If you think your asthma attacks may be triggered by food, start keeping a diet diary. Write down what and when you eat, and see if you find a link to your attacks. Once you suspect a certain food, eliminate it from your diet for five to 14 days, and then reintroduce it to see if it causes a problem.

Once you know a certain food triggers your asthma, the best thing to do is avoid it. But keep in mind the nutrition you get from that food. For instance, if you swear off milk, you need to get calcium from somewhere else. If citrus fruits are your problem, decide where you will get the vitamin C and other antioxidants you need to protect your lungs. A lack of these nutrients can bring on an attack as well.

So blast away at asthma's overall effects by insuring your diet contains plenty of vitamins A, C, and E as well as the minerals magnesium and selenium. All have been proven to help prevent or reduce asthma symptoms.

Jump-start your breathing with a jolt of java

You're probably familiar with a half-dozen reasons why coffee isn't good for you. Well, if you have asthma, here's why you can indulge in a cup or two of java without guilt. The caffeine in your coffee may actually improve your ability to breathe for up to four hours.

A review of six different studies of caffeine and asthma points to that conclusion. The research explains that caffeine is a mild bronchodilator – it opens up swollen airways – and it peps up tired muscles in your respiratory system. It belongs to the same family of chemicals as the drug theophylline, a drug commonly prescribed to treat asthma.

If you're not a coffee drinker, you can get caffeine from soft drinks, tea, cocoa, and chocolate, too. A cup of coffee has about the same amount of caffeine as:

* two diet cokes
* three cups of hot tea
* seven cups of hot chocolate
* 10 Hershey bars

Of course, you have to watch the calories in some of those foods. But they do offer more benefits than just caffeine. The cocao bean contains both theophylline and theobromine, another bronchodilator, and tea is a source of flavonoids that provide antioxidant punch.

But caffeine is also a drug that you can become dependent on, so limit your intake to two drinks a day. More than that can cause withdrawal problems if you cut back suddenly.

CHAPTER 4 *Atherosclerosis*

What is atherosclerosis? This narrowing and thickening of your blood vessels is due to a buildup of cholesterol-rich plaque. This blocks your blood flow, increasing your risk of stroke, heart attack — even death. Researchers now suspect inflammation plays a key role in the development and progression of atherosclerosis.

Who gets it? People with high cholesterol, high blood pressure, and diabetes are at risk. Smoking, obesity, stress, and a lack of exercise also contribute.

What are the symptoms? No early symptoms. Later signs include:

- pain in the chest, arm, jaw, or back
- heart attack
- stroke

Nutrition-packed produce clears arteries

Worried about clogged arteries? Fill up your grocery cart with fruits and vegetables. The produce aisle offers a cornucopia of foods that combat atherosclerosis.

Fruits and vegetables give you plenty of fiber, which lowers cholesterol. They're also loaded with antioxidants that prevent bad cholesterol from becoming oxidized and even more dangerous. On top of that, they taste great. So keep your artery walls clean and prevent blood clots with these scrumptious, nutrition-packed foods.

Chomp cherries. Good things come in small packages. Just look at a cherry. This tiny, sweet fruit contains over 17 compounds to clear away artery-clogging plaque far better than vitamin supplements. These compounds, found in the anthocyanins that give cherries their red color, have even more antioxidant activity than heavyweights, like vitamin C or vitamin E supplements.

Anthocyanins also squash inflammation, which can contribute to atherosclerosis. They work by stopping the enzymes that make prostaglandins, hormone-like substances that cause inflammation and pain. A Michigan State University study found that 20 tart cherries were at least as effective as other painkilling remedies, including aspirin, ibuprofen, and other nonsteroidal anti-inflammatory drugs (NSAIDs). That's why cherries are a popular folk remedy for arthritis and gout.

Dried cherries make a great snack. One dried cherry gives you the same benefits as about eight fresh ones.

Like many fruits and vegetables, cherries also have fiber and potassium to help your heart. Fiber lowers cholesterol, while potassium helps regulate your blood pressure so your heart isn't working overtime. Make room for cherries, whether in jams or juices or just right off the stem.

Guzzle grape juice. A whole grape is greater than the sum of its parts. Both grape skin extract and grape seed extract have a few heart-healthy properties — but together, they're a dynamic duo.

That's why grape juice, made from whole grapes, is an artery-clearing wonder. It protects your artery walls from cholesterol because of several powerful substances.

Quercetin, a flavonoid found in the skin, acts as an antioxidant to prevent LDL cholesterol from collecting on your artery walls. Resveratrol, also found in the skin, thwarts inflammation and blood clots. Meanwhile, procyanidins in the seeds help keep your blood vessels relaxed and exert antioxidant powers of their own.

It's easy to get the benefits of all these substances – just think purple. A recent University of Wisconsin study found that drinking just two glasses of purple grape juice a day helps rejuvenate and protect your arteries.

Munch an apple. Students who bring their teacher an apple are doing more than seeking favor – they're giving the teacher an "A" in heart health.

Apples contain pectin, a soluble fiber that lowers cholesterol. They're also a rich source of quercetin as well as potassium and magnesium, minerals that help keep your blood pressure under control. No wonder a French study has found that eating two apples a day can help prevent and reverse hardening of the arteries.

Try tomatoes, grapes, strawberries, and sweet potatoes. Eat health friendly foods like these to get a variety of nutrients that even the most complete multi-vitamin can't match. Here's a quick look at these four foods that reduce cholesterol build-up in the arteries.

- Tomatoes are chock-full of the carotenoid lycopene, an antioxidant that can slash your risk of atherosclerosis nearly in half. Tomato sauce, soup, and ketchup give you a more concentrated form of lycopene than fresh tomatoes.

- Red seedless grapes are a good source of lutein, a carotenoid that's been shown to combat early atherosclerosis. In recent studies, lutein helped prevent thickening of the carotid artery in the neck, an indication of atherosclerosis. It also reduced inflammation of LDL cholesterol in artery walls.

- Strawberries are loaded with antioxidants, including vitamins C and E, ellagic acid, assorted carotenoids, and anthocyanins. These mighty berries can cut cholesterol levels by 10 percent. So why not toss some into your breakfast cereal?

- Sweet potatoes are crammed with fiber, potassium, beta carotene, folate, and vitamin C to lower your blood pressure and keep your arteries clear.

For variety, and more protection against atherosclerosis, try artichokes, guava, oranges, pomegranate juice, prunes, pumpkin, and rhubarb. Your options are wide open – just like your arteries. Keep your blood flowing to your heart by eating right.

Organic fanatics reap more benefits

When it comes to fighting atherosclerosis, vegetables are great – but organic vegetables are even better.

A recent Scottish study found that soup made with organic vegetables has significantly more salicylic acid than soup made with veggies that aren't organic. Salicylic acid, the active ingredient in aspirin, helps fight inflammation and safeguard your arteries. Look for organic fruits, vegetables, and other products in your grocery store. Thanks to new federal guidelines, it's easier than ever to identify them.

- 100 percent organic – no synthetic pesticides, herbicides, chemical fertilizers, antibiotics, hormones, additives, or preservatives

- Organic – contains 95 percent or more organically produced ingredients

- Made with organic ingredients – at least 70 percent of the product is organic

- If less than 70 percent of the product is organic, the word "organic" can't appear on the front of the package, but it can appear in the list of ingredients.

Healthy fats play starring role

Fats, like many actors, have been typecast. They're always the heavies. But in the ideal script for good nutrition, fats aren't just bad guys. Certain fats can even play the role of hero.

Here's a blockbuster idea for your heart — give these two fats a part in your diet.

Three cheers for omega-3. Fight the triple threat of heart disease with omega-3 fatty acids. They clear clogged arteries, lubricate clumping blood cells, and ease high blood pressure.

And that's not all. These polyunsaturated fats also help regulate your heartbeat and combat inflammation. In a recent Danish study, people with low levels of C-reactive protein, an indicator of inflammation, also had high levels of docosahexaenoic acid (DHA), a specific type of omega-3 fatty acid.

Omega-3 also fights inflammation by countering the inflammatory effects of omega-6, another type of fatty acid. Most people eat a diet overloaded with omega-6, which is found in vegetable oils like soybean or corn oil.

A more balanced ratio of omega-6 and omega-3 will help lessen inflammation, which contributes not only to heart disease but also arthritis, headaches, and asthma. Try to cut down on deep-fried foods and other sources of omega-6 while boosting your intake of omega-3.

Fish, especially fatty fish, is the best source of this amazing nutrient. In fact, the American Heart Association recommends eating two fatty fish meals a week. You'll get the most omega-3 from mackerel, salmon, tuna, and herring, but all fish have some.

Here's something to keep in mind. When buying salmon, you might want to go out of your way for salmon caught in the wild.

Most supermarkets sell farmed salmon, which is much cheaper and available year-round. But recent studies have found that farmed salmon has less omega-3 and more toxins than wild salmon.

Try walnut oil for salad dressings, cooking, baking, or sauteing. Loaded with omega-3, it's a healthy, though pricey, alternative to soybean or corn oils.

You can also find omega-3 in walnuts, which have repeatedly been shown to lower cholesterol. Other sources of omega-3 include flaxseed, wheat germ, and some green leafy vegetables.

Bravo for monounsaturated fats. Feel free to cheer the performance of omega-3, but save some applause for the next act. Monounsaturated fat is no slouch, either. It lowers your bad LDL cholesterol while protecting your good HDL cholesterol.

Olive oil, a great source of monounsaturated fat, has been shown to lower cholesterol and blood pressure and modify the effects of inflammation. Canola oil, avocados, and nuts are other good sources of monounsaturated fat.

Both omega-3 and monounsaturated fatty acids are nutritious stars just waiting to be discovered. Scrub clogged arteries clean by adding these two fats to your diet.

But remember, fat is still fattening. Don't just add more fat to your existing diet. Make sure to cut calories somewhere else. A good strategy would be to trim saturated fats, like red meat, cheese, and butter, and replace them with these healthier, unsaturated fats.

Conquer heart disease with amazing vitamins

You already grew up to be big and strong. But that doesn't mean you should stop taking your vitamins. Whether found in foods or taken as supplements, vitamins can be valuable allies in the war against atherosclerosis. Here's how certain vitamins can help.

Enjoy more E. By preventing the oxidation of LDL cholesterol, vitamin E guards your arteries from plaque build-up – or so the theory goes. Once the hero of heart health, vitamin E's reputation has diminished lately. Several recent studies have found no conclusive evidence that vitamin E provides any benefits to your heart.

But don't dismiss vitamin E just yet. A new Italian study showed that vitamin E was absorbed better when taken with food. People in the small study who took vitamin E with dinner boosted their antioxidant capacity by 14 percent, while those who took the supplement a few hours before lunch showed no change.

On top of that, another recent Italian study found that women who got more vitamin E in their diet had fewer early signs of atherosclerosis.

If you take vitamin E supplements, remember to take them with food. You can also find vitamin E in wheat germ, vegetable oils, nuts, seeds, and some leafy green vegetables. Previous studies have found that vitamin E from food sources was more protective than supplements.

Hit high C. Keeping a stiff upper lip is OK – but the same can't be said of your blood vessels. Loosen up and reach for some vitamin C. This easy-to-find vitamin neutralizes toxic chemicals, called free radicals, that cause hardening of the arteries.

A recent Belgian study showed a link between low levels of vitamin C and peripheral artery disease, a form of atherosclerosis. Vitamin C also counteracts inflammation and boosts levels of beneficial HDL cholesterol. Because of these benefits, Japanese researchers recommend older people get more vitamin C into their diet to stave off atherosclerosis.

In fact, eating foods rich in antioxidants like vitamins C and E reduces your risk of death from many causes, including heart disease, stroke, and cancer. Good sources of vitamin C include citrus fruits like oranges and grapefruits, cruciferous vegetables like broccoli and brussels sprouts, and bright fruits and vegetables like red and green peppers, strawberries, and cantaloupe.

Get the buzz on B's. When you need to stop heart disease dead, summon the killer B's. Folate and other B vitamins swarm through your body to provide maximum protection.

Studies show that people who take folate daily significantly reduce their risk of suffering a heart attack or stroke. Finnish researchers determined that people who got the most folate through their diet were less than half as likely to have a stroke or heart attack as those who got the least.

According to a Chinese study, folate helps get rid of homocysteine, a risk factor for heart disease. It also helps your blood vessels dilate, or widen, so more blood and oxygen can get through.

B vitamins do more than lower your odds of having a stroke. This same vitamin family was also proven to heal stroke damage. Stroke survivors who took a vitamin supplement containing vitamins B12, B6, and folate showed fewer signs of blood vessel damage after three months than those given a vitamin supplement without the B vitamins.

You can find folate in dark leafy greens, legumes, seeds, and enriched breads and cereals. Vitamin B12 shows up in meats, fish, dairy foods, and eggs, while vitamin B6 can be found in greens, legumes, seafood, whole grains, and various fruits and vegetables.

Remember, "B" smart, "C" how much vitamins can help, and give yourself an "E" for effort.

Renovate your food pyramid

Watch out. The familiar USDA Food Pyramid might be just another pyramid scheme.

Harvard researchers determined that following the USDA guidelines didn't have an impact on lowering the risk of chronic diseases. To correct some USDA flaws, they came up with a plan of their own.

This alternate eating plan, based largely on Harvard professor Walter C. Willett's book *Eat, Drink, and Be Healthy*, also promotes fruits, vegetables, and whole grains, but features more specific and logical guidelines.

For example, unlike the USDA pyramid, which lumps all fats together in the "Use sparingly" sliver at the top, the alternate plan distinguishes between good fats and bad fats. The same with carbohydrates and meats. It also includes taking a daily multivitamin.

Another difference – the alternate plan works. Researchers devised the Alternate Healthy Eating Index to measure how well people followed the plan.

Those with the highest scores significantly lowered their risk of cardiovascular disease. Men slashed their risk by 39 percent, while women reduced theirs by 28 percent.

Tap into the benefits of water

Blood is thicker than water. It's also thicker without water. Dehydration can make many risk factors for heart disease, including thick, sticky blood, even worse.

You probably already know you need water to survive. But a recent study suggests that drinking water provides extra benefits for your heart.

Strive for five a day. Dr. Jacqueline Chan and colleagues at Loma Linda University tracked the drinking habits of more than 20,000 people for six years as part of the Adventist Health Study.

People who drank five or more glasses of water a day fared much better against heart disease than those who drank two or fewer glasses of water.

Men in the high-water group slashed their risk of dying from a heart attack by 54 percent, while women cut their risk by 41 percent.

What makes plain old water so good? When you drink water, it becomes absorbed in your blood. This makes your blood less thick – and less likely to clot.

Dump other drinks. Drinking large quantities of other beverages, such as juice, coffee, tea, milk, and alcohol, doesn't help. In fact, it could be harmful.

That's because these beverages thicken your blood and need help being digested. This draws water from your blood into your gut to help dilute these thicker fluids.

In the Adventist study, women more than doubled their risk of dying from a heart attack if they drank lots of beverages other than water. Men boosted their risk by 46 percent.

You don't have to completely eliminate juice, coffee, or other favorite drinks. They can still be a part of a healthy diet. Just limit yourself to no more than two glasses a day.

Meanwhile, focus on increasing your water intake. Here are some quick tips to help you drink enough water each day.

- Drink a glass of water when you get up, during each meal, and before you go to bed to reach your five-glass goal. Fit in more between meals. Don't wait until you're thirsty.

- Wrap five, or more, rubber bands around a plastic mug at the beginning of the day. Remove one with each refill so you know where you stand.

- Take water breaks instead of coffee breaks and drink water instead of cola with lunch.

- Add a splash of fruit juice or a slice of lemon or lime to make plain water more exciting.

Throw your heart a tea party

Does a healthy heart sound like your cup of tea? Pour yourself a cup of this popular hot beverage and find out.

Tea, enjoyed around the world for centuries, can do wonders for your heart and arteries.

Loaded with flavonoids, especially compounds called catechins, tea dilates arteries and improves blood flow. It may also squelch the inflammation associated with atherosclerosis and keep your blood from clotting.

More than one study has determined that drinking one or more cups of tea a day can slash your risk of heart attack in half. Even if you've already had a heart attack, drinking tea may help you live longer.

Most recently, a Japanese study found that drinking tea after a fatty meal prevents your arteries from stiffening.

Penn State University nutrition professor Penny Kris-Etheron brings up another good point. "Since tea, without milk or sugar, contains no calories, it's an ideal way to add antioxidant flavonoids to your diet without increasing your weight," she says.

Fend off clogged arteries with herbs

When the FBI wants to stop a public enemy, it sends out its G-men. To stop atherosclerosis, reach for the herbal version of these special agents.

Remember the four G's – four herbs that improve your heart's health. The first two reduce cholesterol levels, while the third and fourth prevent clogged arteries. All four get the job done.

Garlic. Studies have shown this fragrant kitchen staple lowers cholesterol and blood pressure and prevents blood clots from forming. Garlic also helps fight off infection, which has been linked to inflammation and atherosclerosis.

No wonder garlic has become one of the world's most popular herbs. Many health experts recommend eating 4 grams, or about one clove, a day. Garlic is also available in powdered and pill forms.

Lately, the outlook for "the stinking rose" isn't as rosy. Recent studies are inconclusive about garlic's ability to help your heart. It still seems to lower cholesterol and prevent blood clots in short-term trials, and some studies found it lowered blood pressure, too. However, the studies weren't always set up properly, leaving researchers with more questions than answers about garlic. While the research continues, it won't hurt to add some garlic to your diet.

Ginseng. This ancient herb has been used to treat heart problems for centuries. Sometimes the oldest remedies are the best. Because of a substance called sitosterol, ginseng may lower cholesterol and triglyceride levels. This means a lower risk of clogged arteries and heart disease.

Ginseng acts as an antioxidant and helps keep your blood from clumping. It also revs up your immune system and relieves stress, a factor in heart disease.

You can find ginseng in supplement form. Look for supplements standardized to 4 to 7 percent ginsenosides. Herbal experts recommend taking 100 milligrams (mg) once or twice daily. You can also use a half teaspoon of the root to make a cup of tea.

> **Keep your eyes open. Ginseng also crops up in teas, soft drinks, and even chewing gum.**

Ginger. Your name doesn't have to be Fred to dance around heart disease with this trusty partner. Thanks to antioxidant compounds called gingerols and shogaols, ginger can make anyone footloose and fancy-free.

Ginger helps your body digest fat and may prevent blood clots. A recent Israeli study found that ginger lowers cholesterol and inhibits LDL oxidation in mice. Previous studies showed the same results in rabbits. A 1-inch chunk of fresh ginger will give you the recommended dosage of 2 to 4 grams a day. You can also find ginger supplements in 500 mg capsules. Herbal experts recommend taking three capsules twice daily.

Ginkgo. Remember this. An herb often taken to boost your memory is also great for your circulation. Loaded with antioxidant flavonoids, ginkgo is another powerful herb that single-handedly rids your body of the toxins that cause hardening of the arteries. Ginkgo also widens your blood vessels, improves blood flow, and prevents your blood from clumping.

Your options aren't limited to the four G's. Check out these other herbs that help conquer atherosclerosis.

- Hawthorn is jam-packed with flavonoids to control LDL cholesterol and widen the blood vessels around your heart. It's a good idea to check with your doctor before using this herb. Too much can be toxic.

- Fenugreek contains lots of fiber to help lower bad cholesterol and triglycerides. Use whole or ground fenugreek seeds in cooking. You can find them in an Indian foods market.

- Turmeric has antioxidant and anti-inflammatory powers. It also lowers cholesterol and blocks LDL oxidation. Use some of this spice in your cooking.

Herbs can be great secret agents against atherosclerosis, but don't keep them a total secret. Make sure you tell your doctor you're taking them. Many of these herbs are blood-thinners that can interact with prescription medication, like warfarin, or NSAIDs, like aspirin and ibuprofen.

The latest buzz on garlic supplements

You've heard garlic helps your heart. But helping yourself to the best garlic supplement can be tricky. The key is the amount of allicin, the ingredient that gives garlic its powers. A company called ConsumerLab recently tested 14 garlic products. Here are some of its findings.

- Claims like "allicin-rich" are not necessarily helpful. Some products have less – and some much more – than what they claim

- Some products list the amount of "alliin" instead. Your body converts this to allicin, but you only get about 10 to 50 percent of it.

- Most positive garlic studies used 3,600 to 5,400 micrograms (mcg) of allicin a day. To get that amount from a supplement, you might need to take anywhere from 600 milligrams (mg) to over a gram a day, depending on the allicin yield of the product.

- Enteric coating may help because more allicin will be produced in your gut.

If all this sounds too complicated, remember fresh garlic is always an option. One 4-gram clove gives you 4,000 to 12,000 mcg of allicin – which is plenty.

Super strategies to heal your heart

Spontaneity certainly makes life more exciting. But it's not always the healthiest approach to eating. To make sure your diet leads to a healthy heart, you need a plan. As the slogan goes, failing to plan is planning to fail. Stick with one of these popular and effective diet plans, and you'll get results.

Participate in the Pritikin program. Is this the last diet plan you'll ever need? In less than one month, women and men on this delicious and nutritious plan lost weight without dieting; reduced their cholesterol 21 percent; improved their sense of well being; felt less anxiety, fear, and depression; reduced chest pain by 91 percent; felt renewed energy; and required much less sleep.

The basic elements of this program, which has been around since the 1970s, include a diet low in fat, calories, and salt, as well as moderate exercise. It's great for your blood pressure and cholesterol levels, which play an important role in the development of heart disease.

Opt for the Ornish diet. Another successful program is the well-known Ornish diet. This very low-fat, high-carbohydrate vegetarian diet works in conjunction with exercise and stress management to reverse heart disease.

Do this for four weeks to get rid of plaque and lower cholesterol. It takes at least that long to break bad habits and establish a new, healthy lifestyle.

The longer you stick with it, the better. People who followed Dr. Dean Ornish's regimen for five years reversed the narrowing of their arteries even more than they did after one year. They also had only half as many cardiac events – heart attacks, angioplasties, bypass surgeries, hospitalizations, and deaths – as those who adopted more moderate lifestyle changes.

Approach Atkins with caution. On the other side of the spectrum is the popular Atkins diet. This high-fat, high-protein, low-carbohydrate diet also restricts calories, but lets you load up on traditional dieting outlaws like steak, pork, and eggs.

While this sounds like fun, there are some health issues to consider. Here are some common criticisms and concerns regarding high-protein diets.

- By limiting carbohydrates such as fruits, vegetables, and bread, you force your body to look elsewhere for energy. First, it uses any carbohydrates you have stored, before going after stored protein from your muscles and organs, and then, finally, stored fat.

- You might lose weight, but the high levels of saturated fat and cholesterol increase your risk of heart disease, stroke, and cancer.

- All that protein can affect how your kidneys work, making it potentially dangerous for diabetics with kidney problems.

- The diet is boring and hard to stick with. Once you return to a normal amount of carbohydrates, your weight will probably come back.

In spite of this, a new study at Duke University revealed some surprising results. Not only did people on the Atkins diet lose more weight than those on a standard low-fat, low-calorie diet, they also improved their cholesterol.

Atkins dieters saw their levels of dangerous VLDL (very low-density lipoprotein) cholesterol decrease by 49 percent while their levels of protective HDL cholesterol shot up 8 percent. Compare that with the low-fat dieters who had just a 17-percent decrease in VLDL and a mere 1-percent boost in HDL.

Before you rush out for a fatty steak dinner, remember this is only one small study. Talk with your doctor before drastically changing your diet.

Most experts agree that a low-fat, high-fiber diet, regular exercise, and weight loss — if you're obese — is the best approach to fighting atherosclerosis.

Healthy habits

Eating right isn't the only step in beating atherosclerosis. For more protection, try these lifestyle changes.

- Quit smoking.
- Exercise regularly, even walking helps.
- Lose weight if you're overweight.
- Find ways to cope with stress, such as listening to music or doing yoga.

CHAPTER 5

Breast cancer

What is breast cancer? Breast cancer is uncontrolled growth of abnormal cells in the breast.

Who gets it? Women are far more likely to get breast cancer than men, but men should be aware that it can affect them, too. Breast cancer risk is higher for women over 60, women who have never had children, women who had a first child after 30, and women whose close relatives have had breast cancer.

What are the symptoms?

- lump in or near the breast
- thickened breast tissue or puckered breast skin
- nipple discharge, retraction, or scaliness
- breast pain

Pile on produce to push away cancer

Nibbling a small amount of vegetables each day won't protect you from breast cancer. Eating lots of them may cut your risk in half. Sound like a no brainer? Despite these findings and the fact that lifelong vegetarians may have a slightly lower danger than women on a standard diet, most women still aren't getting their five servings a day.

And eating five or more servings of vegetables and fruits is critical to your overall health, says Melanie Polk, a registered dietician and director of nutrition education at the American Institute for Cancer Research.

"According to surveys, many Americans barely eat two or three servings of vegetables and fruits in the course of a day, and that's not nearly enough to satisfy our nutritional needs," she explains. "Five servings a day is really the minimum. But health experts advise that nine servings should be our goal."And reaching that goal might be easier than you expect.

"Some people might think eating five daily servings of fruits and vegetables is a big challenge," Polk says. "But it is fairly easy to accomplish once you set a goal and realize a standard serving is just one-half cup for most types of fruits and vegetables." What's more, when the five-a-day goal is reached, it takes only a little more effort to gradually, week by week, add a few more servings."

Focus on eating these cancer-crushing foods, and your body will have much of the defense it needs to fight off breast cancer and other diseases.

Head for the cabbage aisle. Cabbage and all its cousins are members of the brassica family, a clan famous for its cancer-fighting abilities. Many cabbage family members prevent cancer with two nutrients called indoles and isothiocyanates.

> For tastier greens, cook them with spices. Add mustard seed to broccoli, marjoram to kale, or dill to brussels sprouts.

Recently, scientists from Finland discovered that the fermentation process used to turn white cabbage into sauerkraut also creates isothiocyanates in the sauerkraut.

Some researchers think you need to eat an awful lot of sauerkraut to get real protection, but you don't have to just eat sauerkraut all day. You can also get cancer defense from these other cabbage family members.

- **Broccoli.** Berkeley scientists say the indole-3-carbinol hiding in those little trees of broccoli may stop the growth of breast cancer cells.

- **Kale.** Dark green kale contains glucosinolates, a chemical that blocks the cancer-forming process. Kale's leaves are also a good source for indoles. If the taste of kale doesn't appeal to you, just switch to its next of kin, collards.

- **Bok choy.** This "Chinese cabbage" has a thick white stem base and big, dark green leaves. Bok choy guards you with its isothiocyanates and pack of indoles.

- **Cauliflower.** Cauliflower's glucosinolates help your body use estrogen safely – and that may reduce your risk. Cauliflower gives you indoles, too. For a sweeter taste, try broccoflower, a bright green version of cauliflower.

- **Brussels sprouts.** Chow down on brussels sprouts to arm your body with indoles and a cancer repelling isothiocyanate called sulphorophane.

Pack in some parsley. Skip out on parsley and you'll miss two anti-cancer nutrients, vitamin C and the flavonoid, apigenin. Canadian research suggests that apigenin may stand in for estrogen. That could mean less circulating estrogen in your body and less breast cancer risk. So eat that parsley garnish or, better yet, add whole parsley to a sandwich or salad.

Sniff out garlic and onions. According to French scientists, eating garlic and onions may be linked with lower breast cancer odds. On top of that, a Penn State study found that selenium and garlic could prevent breast cancer in animals exposed to a strong cancer-causing substance.

> **Want onions that you don't have to chop or peel? Get a pack of frozen onions from the grocery store.**

Garlic and onions both pack a pretty good antioxidant punch, so it's not a bad idea to tuck a few more of them into your diet. Try the minced or powdered versions of onion or garlic to season almost any food. Some folks like to eat onions fresh and raw, but cooked garlic or onions can be tasty, too.

Track your folate. Research shows a lack of folate may raise the odds of breast cancer. Add more folate to your diet to help keep your risk down. It won't be hard because you can easily slip this B vitamin into any meal.

Focus on adding vegetables such as spinach, asparagus, broccoli, collards, lettuce, and corn. At breakfast, try a fortified cereal or orange juice from concentrate. Add lentils, black-eyed peas, or chickpeas (garbanzo beans) to lunch. For a Mexican-style dinner, include black beans, or try chili with pinto beans.

Don't be afraid to pile on the fruits and vegetables each day. Not only is it good for your health, it may just give you the upper hand in the fight against breast cancer.

Crush your risk of breast cancer

A hearty whole grain cereal sprinkled with nutty-tasting flaxseed may help you avoid breast cancer. The fiber in these foods could be the vital ingredient.

Fiber not only gives you that satisfying just-full-enough feeling, but it may also help shrink circulating estrogen levels for women who haven't reached menopause. Less estrogen in your bloodstream could mean less risk of breast cancer. So get more breast-protecting fiber from these appealing foods.

> Try mixing flaxseed into applesauce, yogurt, or hot breakfast cereal for a fiber-filled treat.

Fight back with flaxseed. A small University of Minnesota study showed that eating flaxseed may decrease a kind of estrogen associated with breast cancer. What's more, the researchers suspect that the phytoestrogen lignan might be flaxseed's secret for rooting out risk-raising estrogens. Flaxseeds may be small, but they are the richest source of lignans you can get.

And that's not all. Flaxseeds are an intense source of fiber. A single tablespoon can contain as much as 2.2 grams. If you're trying flaxseed for the first time, start small. Otherwise, you may get gas and indigestion from adding too much fiber at once. Instead, just add

If you're pregnant, taking prescription drugs, or have a serious health condition, ask your doctor before adding flaxseed to your diet.

more flaxseed gradually until you can comfortably eat two tablespoons of flaxseed each day.

Crunch is the key to getting the anti-cancer power of flaxseed. If you swallow flaxseeds whole, your body won't absorb them. They just slip right through your system without doing much good. On the other hand, if you chew your seeds – or buy them already ground – your body can tap into flaxseed's cancer defenses. Look for whole flaxseeds or ground flaxseed meal at your supermarket or local health food store.

Help yourself to whole grains. Study after study shows that whole grains battle cancer. Some experts say whole grains get their cancer-fighting ability from their high fiber content. The refining process strips grains of their nutrient-rich outer layers. But whole grains are processed less so they keep their outer layers and most of their nutrition and fiber.

You can add health-promoting fiber to your diet simply by switching from refined to whole-grain foods. Some people even say whole grain breads and cereals have a richer taste, too. Don't be afraid to branch out from whole wheat products either. Whole grains include hearty whole oats, old-fashioned oatmeal, nutty-flavored brown rice, natural popcorn, and sweet whole grain corn. If you want even more choices, consider these ideas.

- Millet is high in fiber, protein, and magnesium. Look for it in cereals, or try steamed whole millet for yourself. Pet birds love it and you might, too.

- Barley is nearly bursting with fiber. Even the partially refined pearl barely has 5 grams of fiber per cup — and that's after cooking. Potassium-rich barley makes a satisfying breakfast cereal. It is great for soups, too.

- Other grains to try include buckwheat, bulgur, triticale, spelt, teff, and kamut. They may sound strange, but they're well worth getting to know.

Although recommended amounts of fiber range from 21 to 38 grams per day, most Americans only get between 5 and 20 grams daily. Armed with flaxseed and whole grains, you can start getting more of the fiber you need to stay healthy and help keep breast cancer at bay.

New therapy cuts treatment time

A new radiation therapy device may be a first step to shorter treatments and fewer side effects for women with early-stage breast cancer.

Women who have had a cancerous breast lump removed usually need follow-up radiation treatments to kill any remaining breast cancer cells. That could mean up to seven more weeks of pain and unpleasant side effects.

Doctors often supplement breast irradiation with internal radiation therapy, called brachytherapy. This method delivers radioactive "seeds" directly to the cancer site through multiple catheters.

Recently, the Food and Drug Administration (FDA) approved a new brachytherapy device called MammoSite, which delivers all its radiation through just one catheter. Even better, five days of daily treatments may be enough. Researchers hope some women can eventually use it as the sole radiation treatment for early-stage tumors.

Harvest some cancer prevention

A traditional American Thanksgiving dinner could help you prevent breast cancer. But why wait for a holiday? Feast on these festive treats year round, and you may get protection you can be thankful for.

Binge on beta carotene. Pumpkin pie, sweet potato casserole and cooked carrots are not just great Thanksgiving dishes. They're also great sources of beta carotene, a cancer-repelling antioxidant found in foods. In a Johns Hopkins University study, women with the most beta carotene, lycopene, and total carotenoids in their bloodstreams had 50 percent less risk of breast cancer than women with the lowest blood levels of carotenoids.

To boost your beta carotene, eat foods with that beta-carotene orange glow. If you like pumpkin pie, try pumpkin puree and cinnamon mixed into creamy yogurt or a hearty, hot cereal. For a satisfying snack, eat a baked sweet potato with cinnamon and a sliver

> Craving Italian food instead? Eat spaghetti or pizza with tomato sauce for a good dose of lycopene, a cancer-fighting antioxidant.

of butter. You can even jazz up cooked carrots with ground cloves or thyme. Other sources of beta carotene include spinach, broccoli, mango, cantaloupe, and apricots.

Gobble up extra antioxidants. Add cranberry sauce to your Thanksgiving dinner, and you may get more benefits than you expect. A University of Illinois study found that antioxidants in cranberries may stop cancer before it starts. Research from Canada adds that cranberry juice may help prevent breast cancer. On top of that, both cranberries and cranberry juice are sources of cancer-blocking vitamin C. So pile on the cranberry sauce or drink some cranberry juice whenever you like.

If you like your cranberry in a glass, remember that more sweetener can mean less cranberry juice. When buying juice at the supermarket, hunt for the product with the highest percentage of cranberry juice and the least sugar or corn syrup. Pure cranberry juice packs the most nutrient power, but you may have to go to a health food store to get it.

Yet, if you can "strike gold" by finding pure, unsweetened juice, don't worry about the tart flavor. Just sweeten it with carrot juice, and you'll harness the health-building might of vitamin C, cranberry antioxidants, and beta carotene all in one glass!

Go to the citrus bowl. Want more of vitamin C's anti-cancer power? Load your holiday fruit salad with vitamin C-filled citrus fruits. Many citrus fruits also offer antioxidants from flavonoids or beta carotene. What's more, the fiber in citrus may foil cancer, too. To pile protection on your holiday salad, sample slices of orange, tangerine, tangelo, mandarin orange, or even grapefruit. For added vitamin C punch, accent your dish with strawberry, kiwi, papaya, or guava.

Pour on top-notch protection

Breast cancer protection can come from a glass, a carton, or even a mug. Try these refreshing drinks to boost your defenses.

Venture into veggie juices. Research from Johns Hopkins University suggests carotenoids may protect against breast cancer. Carotenoids are remarkable nutritional chemicals. They not only lend red, yellow, or orange color to many fruits and vegetables, but they can also help your body fight diseases, including breast cancer.

That's a good reason to open up a veggie cocktail. Why? Because a single serving of tangy vegetable juice cocktail can give you the extra benefits of four health-promoting carotenoids – alpha carotene, beta carotene, lutein, and lycopene.

What's more, an earlier carotenoid study found that your body may get more alpha carotene and lutein from vegetable juice than from good old-fashioned solid vegetables. So drink up!

Save room for citrus. What puts the orange in oranges and tangerines? Flavonoids. These are more plant-coloring nutrients that can help your body fight off disease. Flavonoids from tangerine juice and orange juice can slow the growth of several types of lab-grown human cancer cells, according to researchers. Of all the flavonoids tested, tangeretin packed the most wallop against cancer cells. Even better, the vitamin C in these citrus juices is an enemy of cancer, too. So help yourself to more orange juice or tangerine juice, and you may just help yourself against cancer, too.

> Looking for tangerine juice? When you shop for orange juice, see if it's shelved nearby, or try the natural foods aisle. You can also check for it in juice blends.

Count on cranberry juice. Scientists have found cancer-fighting compounds hidden in cranberry juice. In fact, research shows this crimson juice may specifically help prevent breast cancer. To get the anti-cancer advantages of cranberry juice, keep this in mind. When cranberry juice drinks include other juices or sweeteners, that means you get less pure cranberry juice – and reduced cancer-busting nutrients.

So pick the bottle with the highest percentage of cranberry juice and the tiniest amounts of sugar or artificial sweeteners. If you're lucky enough to find pure, unsweetened cranberry juice, you'll get the most intense cranberry protection.

Consider the benefits of milk. After a study from Finland tracked nearly 5,000 women for 25 years, the researchers discovered that women who drank more milk lowered their risk of breast cancer. No other dairy product had this effect. Researchers weren't sure why milk worked so well, but they thought the milk's lactose or calcium might be helping behind the scenes.

Recent Harvard studies have stirred up a controversy about milk and breast cancer though. New findings suggest milk may raise the levels of insulin-like growth factor 1 or IGF-1 – a hormone that may be associated with breast cancer risk. On the other hand, researchers also looked at data from the Nurses' Health Study and found that low-fat dairy products, especially milk, may lower breast cancer risk for women who have not reached menopause.

So is milk good for you or bad for you? The Harvard scientists say they need more research to find out whether milk, itself, is the real villain – or just an innocent bystander. Meanwhile, they're not recommending you give it up.

Go for green tea. If you haven't discovered the pleasure of green tea yet, now might be a good time to start. A Boston University research project found that rats given green tea took longer to develop breast tumors than those drinking water. Although the tea-drinking rats developed more tumors, they were smaller and less invasive than those of the other rats.

Other animal studies have supported green tea as a possible cancer fighter, but human studies have not been as positive. Obviously, more research needs to be done. But this beverage is full of polyphenols – another group of disease-resisting nutrients – so the potential is there. It wouldn't hurt to get out your favorite mug and enjoy several cups of green tea each day.

Healthy habits

Have you ever made a New Year's resolution to exercise and lose weight? If you've reached menopause – or even gone past it – keeping that resolution could help you keep away from breast cancer.

Here's why. After menopause, your fat cells, rather than your ovaries, make a form of estrogen. If you have more body fat, you'll make more estrogen. And extra estrogen can boost breast cancer danger.

New research from the Pacific Northwest suggests that one great way to dodge breast cancer is to just keep moving. Scientists discovered that women who lost weight by doing aerobic exercise lowered their estrogen levels – even if they had been sedentary for years. Women who merely did stretching exercises had no such luck.

Try activities such as walking or stationary biking for three to four hours per week, and you'll be exercising like the women in the study. And, like them, you may lower both your estrogen levels and your breast cancer risk.

News flash: HRT and alcohol may double risk

You're trying to lower your breast cancer risk so you eat right, exercise, and try to make healthy choices. Now you have to decide whether to continue hormone replacement therapy (HRT). While you're at it, take a look at your drinking habits. The two together may just double your risk of breast cancer.

Find out the facts. Researchers from the long-running Nurses' Health Study analyzed breast cancer risk for women who drink, use HRT, or do both. They discovered that the women with the lowest breast cancer odds were the ones who avoided HRT and either didn't drink or averaged slightly less than one alcoholic drink per day.

Next, the scientists checked how other women's breast cancer risk stacked up compared to this low-risk group. Here is what their results could mean for you.

- If you use HRT for more than five years, but average just under one alcoholic beverage per day, you probably have 30 percent more risk than the low-risk group.

- If you shun HRT, yet average more than one and a half alcoholic drinks daily, you still have 30 percent more risk than the low-risk group. That's right. The hormone-free drinkers in the study had the same risk as hormone users who drank less.

- If you take HRT for more than five years and also average more than one and a half alcoholic drinks per day, you may have twice as much chance of breast cancer as the low-risk group.

Consider your HRT options. A closer look at the numbers hints that women on HRT may have opportunities to lower breast cancer risk. For example, current hormone users from the study seemed to have a stronger link to breast cancer danger than women who had stopped HRT. That may mean that women who give up HRT start reducing their odds soon after stopping.

On top of that, women who used HRT for under five years showed lower risk than the veteran users who'd broken the five-year mark. So ending HRT before the fifth year may help, too. But if you're considering coming off hormone therapy, check with your doctor first.

Savor each sip. You may be surprised to learn the Nurses' Health Study researchers don't expect you to give up alcohol. Because small amounts of alcohol can be good for your heart, the researchers recommend drinking no more than 10 grams of alcohol each day.

But how much is 10 grams? Assuming that the average 12-ounce can of beer has 12.8 grams of alcohol content, you could have approximately three quarters of a can each day. If you prefer wine, you can safely drink about 3 ounces per day. Check your wine glass size to figure out how full to fill it.

Follow these guidelines and you may help protect your heart and fend off breast cancer, too.

CHAPTER 6

Cataracts

What are cataracts? They are a clouding of the lens in one or both eyes.

Who gets them? More than half the people over age 65 have some degree of cataract development. Natural aging is the most common cause. Exposure to ultraviolet light can boost cataract risk. Smoking and diabetes raise the chances of some types of cataracts, too.

What are the symptoms?

- cloudy or blurred vision
- problems with a halo or haze around lights
- poor or distorted color perception
- greater sensitivity to light

Chase off cataracts with two C's

Want to defend your eyes from aging, eye disease, and cataracts? Remember the two C's – vitamin C and carotenoids.

"C" your way to prevention. Studies show vitamin C may help prevent cataracts. For example, in one test group of 4,000 older adults, those who got more vitamin C had a lower chance of cataracts. New research found that women under 60 who averaged 362 milligrams (mg) of vitamin C per day had 57 percent less cataract risk than women who downed 140 mg daily.

The researchers also discovered that women of any age who took vitamin C supplements for 10 years or longer shrunk their cataract odds by 60 percent compared to those who took no supplements.

Vitamin C may have also reduced cataract risk for people in Spain's Valencia region, according to research published recently in the *Journal of Nutrition*. People living in Valencia eat a diet high in citrus fruits and vitamin C, says Dr. Maria Pastor-Valero, the study's lead researcher from the Faculty of Public Health at the University of São Paulo in Brazil.

"The main crops of citrus fruits in the Valencia region are oranges, tangerine, and lemon," Pastor-Valero explains. "These, along with peppers used in our paella, potatoes and some green vegetables, and legumes like lettuce, spinach, cauliflower were the main sources of vitamin C in the population who participated in our study."

In fact, Valencians participating in the study averaged around 157 mg of vitamin C per day. That's more than 60 mg higher than the recommended dietary allowance (RDA) for men and nearly twice the recommended value for women.

Pastor-Valero believes the study findings may be useful in preventing cataracts, but that's not all. They could also affect the RDA for vitamin C.

"These recommendations were established to prevent diseases due to vitamin deficiencies, like scurvy, Pastor-Valero says. "Recent research results on chronic diseases (cardiovascular etc.) and antioxidants seems to suggest that these should be higher."

To sample a sweet orange with bright red flesh, try a Blood orange. The red coloring comes from the flavonoid anthocyanin.

To protect your eyes with vitamin C, try eating citrus like the Valencians. You may be surprised at how many citrus varieties you have to choose from. For example, oranges you can try include Navel, Valencia, Hamlin, and Pineapple. You can also pick up vitamin C from the following foods.

- sweet red peppers (1 cup) – 283 mg

- papaya (one raw fruit) –188 mg

- sweet green peppers (1 cup) – 133 mg

- kiwi (1 medium fruit) – 75 mg

- orange (one raw fruit) – 70 mg

- cauliflower (1 cup, boiled) – 55 mg

- kale (1 cup, boiled) – 53 mg

- tangerine (one raw fruit) – 26 mg

Remember that vitamin C may also slash your risk of cancer, halt heart disease, improve your energy level, and relieve arthritis, so be sure to get plenty of this valuable vitamin.

Look into lutein and zeaxanthin. It's no secret that the plant coloring agents called carotenoids can be good for your eyes, but which ones do you need? One Harvard study found that men who ate high amounts of lutein and zeaxanthin seemed less likely to develop cataracts. Broccoli and spinach were particularly helpful.

Another study showed that nonsmoking women who got more carotenoids and folate might have lower odds of posterior subcapsular cataracts, the kind that disable your vision the most.

Fortunately, some of the foods already loaded with lutein and zeaxanthin are also good sources of vitamin C. Get this triple pack of sight-saving nutrients from broccoli, brussels sprouts, turnip greens, collards, spinach, or kale. Get bonus lutein and zeaxanthin from corn, corn meal, romaine lettuce, Japanese persimmons, or zucchini.

For more information on these super eye-saving carotenoids, see *Slash AMD risk in half* on page 185.

Focus on 6 super sight savers

You should also remember three Bs and "PEA" to help you see. Sure, that sounds strange, but it's a good way to focus on the six nutrients that can help you avoid nuclear cataracts – the kind of cataract that blocks off the center of your vision.

So what are "three Bs and PEA"? The three Bs are vitamins B1, B2 and B3 while PEA stands for Protein, vitamin E, and vitamin A. Researchers say that people who are deficient in these nutrients are more likely to get nuclear cataracts. You can defend against deficiency and vision loss at the same time when you know what foods to eat.

> **Blurred faces, dull colors, and light sensitivity could mean you have cataracts. But medications can cause these symptoms, too. If you're not sure how a drug affects your vision, ask your doctor.**

Try trail mix for thiamin. You can be on the go and still get your eye-protecting thiamin. Just be sure to take along a bag of tropical trail mix. Its mixture of nuts and fruits is full of thiamin, which is another name for vitamin B1. If you like hearty food, you can easily get plenty of thiamin. Just eat lots of nuts, beans, whole grain products, raw oat bran, pork, and brown rice. Adults need 1.1 to 1.2 milligrams (mg) of vitamin B1 each day.

Eat eggs for riboflavin. Did you celebrate December holidays with riboflavin last year? If you drank some eggnog, you probably did. Eggnog contains riboflavin, the second of the three Bs. Of course, you probably don't want to drink eggnog year round. So be sure to eat foods like milk, eggs, meat, chicken, and shiitake mushrooms. For convenient snacks full of vitamin B2, try these:

- ready-to-eat breakfast cereals
- plain yogurt sweetened with your favorite fruit juice

Adults need at least 1.1 mg of vitamin B2 each day. In fact, men should get 1.3 mg.

Make meat and potatoes for niacin. When you think of niacin — vitamin B3 — think "main course." Just as niacin can protect the center of your vision, it is often the centerpiece of your meals, too. It doesn't matter whether you're a "meat and potatoes man," a chicken lover, or a tuna fan. Niacin is in all those foods. You can even get your niacin from liver if that's what you like.

> If you decide to get your niacin from meat and potatoes, you'll get even more if you add mushrooms to the meat and go for a whole, baked potato.

For convenience, check the labels on ready-to-eat breakfast cereals. Scan the nutrition listing for either niacin or vitamin B3. Keep in mind that men need around 16 mg per day, but women only need 14 mg.

Chow down on chicken for protein. You can have your protein and eat healthy, too. Chicken, turkey, and fish are high in protein. They're the kinds of foods that can let you eat light while protecting your sight.

But what if you're a vegetarian? You can get protein from any dish that combines grains and legumes. Because the legumes group includes both beans and peanuts, even whole grain bread with peanut butter gets the job done. If you want something a little wilder, try the Cajun dish red beans and rice. Some people say you can have good luck year round if you remember to have black-eyed peas with rice on New Year's Day — and that could mean good luck for your eyesight, too.

For a protein-rich snack that's portable and meat-free, stick with creamy delicious yogurt.

Pick a papaya for vitamin E. Unlikely as it seems, the lusciously sweet papaya can be a good source for vitamin E. But you also have a whole menu's worth of other choices as well. To eat your required 15 mg per day, try nutty-tasting brown rice, fiber-packed wheat germ, healthy sunflower seed oil, or hearty whole-grain flours. For convenient snacks, sample these:

- sunflower seeds

- canned juice pack peaches

- almonds

- fortified cereal

- peanut butter

Munch on mangoes for vitamin A. Eat a single mango, and you'll get more than 400 micrograms (mcg) of sight-saving vitamin A. That's a good start on the 900 mcg men need daily, and an even better start on the 700 mcg recommended for women. Mix it into a fruit salad, or whip up a delicious smoothy for an easy way to enjoy this exotic fruit.

Of course, you may not want to eat a mango every day to help fill your vitamin A quota. Any of the following foods will do – turnip greens, beef (including liver), canned pumpkin, cooked carrots, baked sweet potato, and spinach. For a convenient snack, nibble on:

- dried apricots

- raw carrots

- sweet red peppers

So when you're thinking about eye health, remember the foods that will give you the 3 Bs and PEA. Keep these nutrients in sight, and you'll have better odds of good vision for years to come.

Healthy habits

For extra eye protection, try these strategies:

- Avoid drinking alcoholic beverages. Drinking every day can raise your cataract odds by 31 percent.

- If you smoke, quit as soon as you can. When compared to nonsmokers, you are up to three times more likely to get cataracts if you smoke.

- Protect your eyes by wearing sunglasses when outside. Make sure the label on the glasses clearly states that they will protect your eyes from nearly all ultraviolet (UV) light.

- Although two years of hormone therapy may lower cataract risk by as much as 20 percent if you're past menopause, new studies have seriously questioned the benefits of long-term HRT. Talk with your doctor about hormone therapy, but be sure to consider other eye-protecting strategies, too.

Cancel out cataracts

Add more selenium to your diet while subtracting salt, and you'll be doing "mineral math" – the kind of arithmetic that may help preserve your eyesight.

Add selenium for defense. Selenium isn't just another mineral. It's also an essential antioxidant for your eyes.

Why do your eyes need antioxidants? Both free radicals and ultraviolet light from the sun can cause cell damage in your eyes. That can lead to eye disease and eyesight problems. Antioxidants are especially suited to fight cell damage and free radicals. Like your own personal SWAT team, they stand ready to defend your eyes. They may also help you avoid the conditions that lead to cataracts.

Selenium is just one of the antioxidants your eyes adore. It works closely with another antioxidant, glutathione. Both selenium and glutathione should normally be present in your eyes – right where they can best defend against cataracts. To make sure you keep an eye full of antioxidants, eat the foods that are loaded with these powerful protectors.

> **Boiling vegetables reduces their natural selenium content. Instead try steaming, sautéing or microwaving.**

To help your body pick up more selenium, cut back on sugar, choose whole grains instead of refined ones, and cook your vegetables lightly. Seek your selenium from Brazil nuts, broccoli, cabbage, celery, cucumbers, and lean meats. And if you're worried about the fat in Brazil nuts, just go easy on them. You only need one or two whole nuts to get enough selenium.

But don't leave your selenium to work alone. Get extra glutathione from raw asparagus, fresh avocado, potatoes, and raw spinach.

Subtract salt for healthier eyes. Too much salt in your diet can push up your blood pressure and interfere with the blood vessels in your eyes. In fact, Australia's Blue Mountains Eye study reported that people who ate 3,000 milligrams (mg) of salt each day were twice as likely to get cataracts as people who ate only 1,000 mg. What's more, Italian scientists found that people who eat the most salt and fat have a higher cataract risk.

So do your eyes a favor, and try to eat less than 2,400 mg of salt per day. If you have high blood pressure, stay below 2,000 mg. Don't think that low-salt eating means boring meals, though. Instead, jazz up familiar foods and limit your salt intake with these ideas.

- Experiment with new ways to season food. You'll be astonished at all your options. Sample spices, seasoning mixes, herbal salt substitutes, sea vegetable or seaweed powders, or even tangy lemon juice.

- Don't add salt to food when you cook it.

- Avoid fast foods.

- Check processed foods by reading the sodium content on labels.

- Keep one or more shakers of your favorite spices or season mixes on the table, so you'll have tasty and convenient alternatives to salt.

Now that you see how mineral math works, add it to your lifestyle. It may just help you subtract cataracts for good.

Tasty ways to head off cataracts

Can you use two more ideas for preventing cataracts? Try these tasty tips.

- **Turn on to turmeric.** Traditionally a spice for curry dishes, turmeric has a new claim to fame – curcumin. Curcumin is a natural antioxidant in turmeric. When researchers fed curcumin to rats, the rats were more resistant to cataracts. Throw some spicy turmeric in your dishes, and see what it does for you.

- **Substitute olive oil for heavier fats.** Saturated fats, such as butter, lard, and hydrogenated vegetable shortenings can raise your risk of cataracts. Use olive oil instead, and get a light taste of what's good for your eyes.

CHAPTER 7

Colds & flu

What are colds and flu? They are infections caused by viruses, not bacteria. A cold usually lasts only a few days. But it takes most people a week or two to recover from the flu, or influenza. Unfortunately, some people develop life-threatening complications from the flu, like pneumonia.

Who gets these infections? Viruses are continually changing over time. This makes people susceptible throughout their lives. Those with immune systems weakened by stress are especially at risk.

What are the symptoms?

- Runny nose, sneezing, coughing, and a sore throat
- Low-grade fever for colds, high-grade fever for the flu
- Fatigue and muscle aches for the flu

New twist on staying healthy

Want to cut your chances of getting a cold or the flu this season? Eat breakfast. Professor Andy Smith of Cardiff University directed a study of 100 people in Wales. He found that people who had fewer colds were more likely to eat breakfast. And they weren't just healthy because they got up early, he points out "breakfast is associated with a general healthy lifestyle, but we controlled for this and [still saw] the breakfast effect."

Take his advice and give colds and flu the cold shoulder with a morning bite. Here's a mouth-watering menu to get you started.

- a glass of orange juice
- a quarter of a cantaloupe, cut into chunks

- a cup of low-fat yogurt or a glass of low-fat milk fortified with live yogurt cultures

- a bowl of whole-grain cereal with low-fat milk, or two slices of whole wheat toast

Start with vitamin C. While vitamin C may not prevent a cold, research shows it might shorten the length of time you suffer from cold symptoms. You can get plenty of vitamin C from traditional breakfast fare, like orange juice, cantaloupe, grapefruit, and strawberries. And when you're tired of these, try tangerines, pomegranate juice, mangoes, and guavas.

> To boost your immune system, Dutch researchers recommend eating more when you have a viral infection and less when you have a bacterial infection.

Add more live cultures. Studies show that the live cultures found in yogurt could improve your health. These cultures, or healthy bacteria, not only encourage the growth of other friendly bacteria in your intestines, they also have a reputation for boosting your immune system. In a study of 571 children in day-care centers in Finland, those given milk fortified with live cultures had fewer colds. And in a group of older adults, those drinking milk containing live cultures had stronger immune systems.

You may have heard you shouldn't drink milk when you have a cold because it increases the amount of mucus you produce, but studies show milk doesn't affect mucus at all. In fact, researchers say drinking milk, even without live cultures, can improve your immune system and help you fight off colds.

Try cereal for selenium. Getting enough selenium is usually not something you have to worry about since it's abundant in grains. But if your levels are low, your bout with the flu could be much worse. In one study, rats deficient in selenium developed a particularly vicious form of the flu.

So get a head start on selenium with a bowl of whole-grain cereal in the morning. If you eat the recommended grain and meat servings a day, you should be getting all the selenium you need to stay healthy.

5 ways to relieve the discomfort

There was a reason your mother rushed to the teapot when you came home with a cough. Recent medical findings support the 'hot cuppa' as your first line of defense against a cold.

Hyssop. Though it might not be related to the hyssop of the Bible, *hyssopus officinalis* has been recommended for centuries as a decongestant. Drink it as a tea to loosen phlegm or gargle with it to soothe a sore throat. Make your own tea by steeping one to two teaspoons of the dried leaves and flowers in boiling water for about 10 minutes, or buy ready-made tea bags at a health food store. For an extra touch of flavor, add a little honey to this healing brew.

Ginger. This fragrant herb can help rid your body of viruses. Gently simmer three to four slices of fresh ginger root in a pint of hot water for 10 to 30 minutes to make a refreshing and soothing remedy.

Pineapple juice and honey. All that coughing and hacking can leave your throat feeling scratchy and sore. Just mix together 8 ounces of warm pineapple juice with two teaspoons of honey for a delicious, soothing drink.

> Try a zinc nasal gel to shorten a cold's duration and reduce the symptoms. You can start treatment up to 48 hours after you first feel a cold coming on.

Chicken soup. Health experts finally caught on to the healing power of chicken soup. Researchers discovered that the hot liquid moistens and clears your nasal passages and soothes your sore throat. It can also relieve symptoms of an upper respiratory tract infection by reducing inflammation. To make your own medically proven home remedy, add some garlic, celery, parsnips, onions, sweet potatoes, carrots, turnips, and parsley to your homemade chicken broth.

Water. Most importantly, drink plenty of water to replace the fluid you are losing. Water will also keep your throat lining moist and supple so it won't crack and let viruses in. Drink eight glasses a day, enough to turn your urine almost clear.

Try herbs to calm your symptoms

New strains of cold and flu viruses appear every year, but with these herbs in your arsenal, you may be able to fight them off.

Elderberry. If your temperature is rising, cool it down with an extract made from the flowers and berries of this ancient bush. Take it when you have the flu to reduce congestion and help you sweat your fever away.

Naturalists also think an extract from the fruit can ward off the flu naturally by making your cells invincible to viruses. Since the leaves and stem of this plant are toxic, herbal experts recommend using only commercially prepared capsules, tablets, or liquid extracts and taking them as directed.

Echinacea. This herb is widely used in Europe to stop colds in their tracks. Though recent research has been contradictory, it has a long history of resisting viral attacks and strengthening the immune system. Many herbalists recommend taking echinacea extract at the first signs of a cold. You may get relief from the stuffy, sneezy, drippy symptoms in only 24 hours.

Echinacea seems most effective when taken sparingly, and it should never be used for more than eight weeks. Don't use this herb if you are allergic to members of the daisy family, or if you have an autoimmune condition like multiple sclerosis.

Thyme. The same herb that seasons your food can relieve congestion. Steep about one teaspoon of this dried herb in a cup of warm water and drink it three times a day. Add honey to soothe your throat.

Marshmallow root. Though not related to the soft, sweet candy you roast at a bonfire, marshmallow root has the gummy texture and slight sweetness of candy. The preparations made from this root can soothe an irritated throat and calm a cough. You can find marshmallow as a liquid extract, powdered root, dried leaves, capsules, and tablets. It's also an ingredient in some cough medicines.

Horehound. A member of the mint family, this herb has a place of honor at the Jewish Passover table. What's more, it has been used for centuries to relieve coughs and congestion. To make a tea, steep one teaspoon of the dried leaves in a cup of boiling water for about 10 minutes. Drink it four or five times a day to clear your sinuses and soothe your cough. If you have an ulcer or gastroesophageal reflux disease (GERD), try another remedy. Horehound activates the digestive juices, and it could worsen your symptoms.

Eucalyptus. The next time a cold kicks in, think like a koala. Eucalyptus, their favorite food, can help ease congestion. Add a few drops of the essential oil to a bowl of steaming water. Cover your head with a towel and inhale the vapors. Your nose might feel stuffier for about a half hour, but be patient. You'll soon be breathing with ease. Eucalyptus thins and loosens mucus so it's easier to cough up. If you prefer a tea, steep one or two teaspoons of leaves in a cup of water for 10 minutes, then strain. You can drink two or three cups a day. Don't use eucalyptus if you have liver problems or inflammation of the stomach or intestines.

Remember, herbs are nature's drugs, but they can interfere with prescription medicines. Check with your doctor before treating yourself with any herb.

Healthy habits

Here are some tips to keep you healthy and save you trips to the doctor this winter.

Get a flu shot. Unless you are allergic to eggs, you should get a flu shot if you are over 50 or have a chronic condition. Because viruses are constantly changing, you must get a flu shot every year. For best results, be well-rested and relaxed. If you're under stress, your body won't respond properly to the vaccine.

Wash your hands religiously. Navy recruits lathered up five times a day and watched their rate of respiratory illness drop by 45 percent. Wash vigorously with regular soap and water for 15 to 20 seconds, long enough to sing the famous "Happy Birthday" song, then rinse.

Work out wisely. Regular exercise can help keep your immune system strong. But if you have a fever, sore muscles or joints, vomiting, diarrhea, or you are coughing up mucus, wait until the infection runs its course before you start exercising again.

If your flu symptoms just won't go away, check for evidence of a tick bite. You could have Lyme disease.

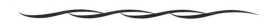

CHAPTER 8

Colon cancer

What is colon cancer? This uncontrolled growth of cells occurs in the tissues of the colon, or large intestine.

Who gets it? The risk of colon cancer increases with age and is most common in those with a personal history of polyps in the colon or rectum, those suffering from ulcerative colitis or other colon disorders, as well as those with a family history of colon cancer. A high-fat, high-calorie, low-fiber diet is also associated with an increased risk of colon cancer.

What are the symptoms? A change in bowel movements (frequency, size, or shape of stools), diarrhea or constipation, blood in the stool, abdominal discomfort, unexplained weight loss, fatigue, and vomiting.

Downsize fats to fight cancer

If you regularly super-size an already high-fat meal from fast-food restaurants, you are putting your health at risk.

"The current American diet can provide more fat on a daily basis than a human being was ever meant to handle," says Dr. David Mangelsdorf, of the University of Texas Southwestern Medical Center at Dallas. As a result, cancers of the colon and rectum are much higher in the United States than in Japan, where a low-fat diet is the norm.

No one is quite sure why fat increases cancer risk. But Mangelsdorf and his fellow researchers believe lithocholic acid, produced as the body processes cholesterol, may be at least part of the reason.

"Lithocholic acid is highly toxic, and it builds up in a high-fat diet," Mangelsdorf says. "We don't know how it causes cancer, but it is known to cause cancer in mice, and people with colon cancer have high concentrations of it."

In addition to watching your fat intake, here are some other ways to protect yourself against colon cancer.

Potato chips, French fries, and other starchy foods fried at high temperatures contain considerable amounts of acrylamide, a possible cancer-causing compound. That's one more reason to choose healthier, low-fat snacks.

Avoid prime protein. European researchers found that red meat, and processed meat in particular, increases the risk of colon cancer. Other studies have connected well-done – especially grilled – meats to colon cancer, as well.

You might replace at least some of the red meat in your diet with broiled fish or baked chicken or turkey breast. Beans are also a good alternate source of protein.

Drink low-fat milk. The lactose, or sugar, in milk seems to protect your colon with healthy bacteria. But go slow on other dairy products. Cheese, buttermilk, and butter may slightly raise your risk of colorectal cancer.

Be choosy about oils. To follow a low-fat diet, you would naturally use oils in moderation. Research, however, shows olive oil may be protective against colon cancer. Corn and safflower oil, on the other hand, may increase your risk.

Battle cancer with the pick of the crop

Fruits, vegetables, and grains may be your most important weapons in the war on cancer. Whether it's due to their antioxidants, their fiber, or some combination of nutrients, the

National Cancer Institute says eat more servings of foods like these every day.

Citrus fruits. Squeeze lots of oranges, tangerines, lemons, and limes into your daily menu. Their antioxidant-rich juice and pulp help shield you against cancers of the colon, stomach, lung, esophagus, prostate, mouth, and larynx.

Black raspberries. These nutritious berries may be scarce but you're going to want to hunt them down. A recent study found black raspberries had 40 percent more antioxidant activity than strawberries and 11 percent more than blueberries.

They contain beta carotene, vitamins C and E, folate, anthocyanins, phenols, and calcium – all helpful in preventing cancer.

Curry dishes can be dynamite against colon and other cancers. The punch comes from curcumin, the active ingredient in turmeric, the spice that gives curry powder its yellow color.

Cabbage. This inexpensive, ultra low-calorie vegetable has ultra high cancer-fighting nutrients. Researchers say it prevents cancer of the colon, brain, breast, stomach, bladder, and lung.

Tomatoes. Fresh tomato slices may perk up a sandwich, but ounce for ounce, there's more cancer-fighting lycopene in the tomato sauce on your pasta or pizza.

Black beans. These dark legumes are high in resistant starch, the indigestible kind that helps fend off colon cancer. All beans are also high in the B vitamin folate, which is especially protective to those with a history of colon cancer.

Spinach. Folate and the antioxidant lutein give spinach a double crack at colon cancer. Other nutrient-rich green vegetables, like kale and broccoli, are also good food choices.

> The antioxidant power of oregano, dill, thyme, rosemary, and other herbs helps fight many cancers. It's best to use fresh since they are more potent than dried.

Whole grains. Oat and whole wheat breads — whether plain or toasted — are good for your colon. White bread, on the other hand, has only one-fourth the fiber. Rye, another good choice, improves bowel movements and may reduce cancer-causing compounds in your colon. Eat corn and barley for their resistant starch.

Not all plant-based foods are your colon's friend, however. Digestible carbohydrates — sugar, white flour, and other highly processed starches — increase cancer risk. In one study, women who ate the most non-fiber carbohydrates increased their risk of colon cancer almost seven times over that of women who ate the least amount. Men who ate the most doubled their risk of cancer of the rectum.

Healthy habits

Follow these suggestions and cut your risk of colon cancer.

- Exercise 30 to 60 minutes a day.
- Lose weight if you are overweight.
- Drink plenty of water every day.
- Ask your doctor about taking a daily baby aspirin.
- Don't smoke.
- Limit alcohol.
- Get regular screenings for colon cancer.

CHAPTER 9 *Constipation*

What is constipation? Constipation is having infrequent or hard to pass bowel movements.

Who gets it? It often affects people who eat a low-fiber diet and get little exercise, as well as those with certain health conditions, including Parkinson's disease, irritable bowel syndrome, diabetes, and depression. People taking certain medications and those who become dependent on laxatives are also prone to constipation.

What are the symptoms?

- infrequent bowel movements
- hard, dry stool
- straining during bowel movements
- abdominal bloating and discomfort

Loosen up with prunes

Old-fashioned prunes, thanks to modern marketing strategy, now have a newfangled name – "dried plums." But whatever you call them, these wrinkled fruits are still one of the best natural laxatives around.

Prunes provide fiber plus other natural laxative ingredients that work together in your digestive tract to keep you regular. Eat them plain out of the box, or put chopped prunes on hot or cold cereals. Use "dried plums" instead of raisins in oatmeal cookies, or stir them into pancake batter.

If you want to replace ground beef with ground turkey in your meatball recipe but find it's too dry, prunes can help out there, too. Just mix in a couple of teaspoons of prunes – pureed with a little hot water in a blender or food processor – per pound of ground turkey.

Need fiber but don't like prunes? Try figs, peaches, carrots, cabbage, beans, seeds, and whole grains.

Hemorrhoid helpers

You can prevent painful hemorrhoids with these simple recommendations.

- Eat high-fiber foods.
- Drink lots of water to soften stools.
- Don't sit too long on the toilet.
- Get plenty of exercise.
- Lose weight if you are overweight.

If you already have hemorrhoids, avoid eating spicy foods, like hot chilies, that might cause pain.

Start or stop bowel action – naturally

Apples – nutritious, low in calories, and fat-free – are plentiful today. But in ancient Greece they were rare. As a special treat, newlyweds shared one apple on their wedding night.

It may be less romantic, but an apple is also a food that keeps you regular. It helps you conquer constipation and diarrhea. With 4 or 5 grams of fiber, a plain raw apple, including the skin, eases constipation.

For diarrhea, try applesauce or a baked apple without the peel. The pectin, a soluble fiber, firms up watery stool.

Healthy habits

These suggestions should help you keep bowel movements regular and comfortable.

- Eat slowly.
- Exercise frequently.
- Drink plenty of liquids.
- Keep regular bathroom habits.
- If you need a laxative, try herbal remedies containing ingredients like flaxseed, senna, psyllium, or castor oil. You can also mix honey into a glass of warm water or drink carbonated water.
- Talk to your doctor or pharmacist about medications that may be causing constipation.
- If you take a multi-vitamin, choose one without iron.
- Relax. Try biofeedback or meditation for stress relief.

CHAPTER 10 *Depression*

What is depression? This medical condition affects mood, thoughts, physical health, and behavior. It's a result of a combination of genetics and psychological and medical factors. Symptoms are linked to brain chemical changes.

Who gets it? One in four seniors with chronic health problems suffer from depression. Usually, the specific cause is unknown, but it can be triggered by certain medications, stress, or major life changes like the death of a loved one.

What are the symptoms?

- feelings of sadness, guilt, irritability, or hopelessness
- trouble concentrating and making decisions
- major changes in appetite, weight, or sleeping habits
- loss of interest in activities
- in extreme cases, thoughts of death or suicide

Blast the blues with feel-good foods

Even mild mood changes can be linked to bad eating habits. Feelings of depression are sometimes early symptoms of nutritional deficiencies, especially in older adults. This puts food on the front lines of the war on depression.

Bust those blahs with B's. B vitamins are essential to your health, but many seniors don't get enough of them. Deficiencies in vitamins B12 and B6, folate, and thiamin have all been linked to high rates of depression.

Women need to pay special attention. If you have low levels of vitamin B12, you double your risk for severe depression. In fact, a recent study found that one in four seriously depressed women were B12 deficient.

But don't despair – eat beef, turkey, and chicken liver; shellfish, salmon; sardines; and trout. Just remember the National Academy of Sciences says almost one-third of seniors can't absorb the vitamin B12 in food. They suggest also eating foods fortified with this nutrient – like many commercially prepared cereals – or supplementing.

A baked white potato packs close to half the B6 you need in a day. And a 3-ounce chicken breast gives you another third of that daily quota.

Vitamin B6 also helps balance certain brain chemicals, keeping your emotions on an even keel. Not getting enough of this nutrient could cause or worsen depression. Seek out foods like liver, seafood, legumes, whole grains, and fortified cereals.

Folate seems to fight that low feeling, too, perhaps by affecting how your brain uses dopamine and serotonin, two natural chemicals that influence mood. Folate is easy to find in fortified breads and cereals, legumes, seeds, and dark green leafy vegetables.

Depression may also be a sign of a thiamin shortage. This B vitamin is essential to how your body uses energy. So it makes sense that whole grains, nuts, meat, legumes, and other thiamin-rich foods could help fend off black moods. A 3-ounce pork chop will give you most of your thiamin requirements for the day.

Up your mood with omega-3. Docosahexaenoic acid (DHA) and eicosapentaenoic acid (EPA) – two kinds of omega-3 fatty acids – could have lots to do with depression. Too little DHA in your body can mean too little serotonin, that important feel-good brain chemical. EPA, on the other hand, shows promise for treating some mental disorders like schizophrenia.

Fish is without question the best natural source for omega-3, followed closely by flaxseed and canola oils, wheat germ, soybeans, and nuts. Eat fatty fish regularly, and you could protect yourself from many serious illnesses. Just two servings of fish each week will bolster your body against depression as well as heart attack, stroke, diabetes, and cancer. Experts suggest getting about 10 ounces of fish weekly to give your body all the omega-3 it needs.

See the bright side with C. This mighty vitamin is vital in making serotonin. That means running low can leave you feeling tired and sluggish. Liven up your life by drinking a glass of orange juice or tossing slices of fresh red and green peppers in your salad. Citrus fruits, dark green leafy vegetables, and other brightly colored fruits and veggies are also solid sources of this mood-lifting vitamin.

Iron out ill moods. Just as certain vitamin deficiencies may trigger depression, so could some mineral shortages. Over two billion people suffer from iron-deficient anemia, a condition that can make you depressed, tired, and unable to concentrate. To ward it off, get your daily iron from dark meat, legumes, leafy green vegetables, and fortified cereals. See your doctor if you think you're anemic. She can test you, treat you, and have you feeling better in no time.

> **Vitamin C helps your body absorb iron. Laying a slice of tomato on your sandwich, for instance, will make the most out of iron in the bread.**

Smile again with selenium. This essential mineral could put a grin on your face. People with healthy amounts of selenium in their bodies tend to be cheerful and confident, while those with too little can become grumps. Since it's a natural part of many foods like beef, seafood, poultry, mushrooms, whole wheat, and sea vegetables you should have no trouble getting all the selenium you need.

Manage your moods with magnesium. Low moods, tiredness, confusion, and loss of appetite are symptoms of depression, but they may also be signs of a magnesium deficiency. Women need about 320 milligrams (mg) a day of this mineral, and men need 420 mg.

A cup of Kellogg's bran cereal with raisins for breakfast puts you on track with over 80 mg of magnesium, while a cup of cooked spinach with your dinner keeps you going with almost 160 mg. Whole grains are rich sources of this mineral, but refined grains provide little. Nuts, legumes, seafood, and dark leafy greens all pack a powerful magnesium punch.

Depression is a serious illness – you can't treat it with just diet. While eating the proper nutrients can lower your risk of depression and speed your recovery, don't try to take on this illness alone. Look to your doctor and loved ones for help, and consider medications if your doctor recommends them.

Friends + food = a better mood

Loneliness can be downright depressing. Turn meal-time into friend-time by gathering with family and neighbors around nutritious, mood-lifting foods. You'll eat well and be with people you care about – just what you need to beat the blues.

- Get together with your church group or other club once a week for a potluck dinner.

- Don't cook for one. Make enough for several people and invite them to join you.

- Make holidays and birthdays count. Gather with loved ones every chance you have.

Now wow your friends and wipe out depression with this delicious meal.

- Bake salmon filets for uplifting omega-3 fatty acids.

- Serve them on a bed of steamed spinach for a healthy dose of magnesium, B6, and folate.

- Add black beans on the side to boost your thiamin as well as your iron.
- Toss a fresh salad with mushrooms for selenium, and broccoli and tomatoes for vitamin C.

St. John's wort: help or hoax?

St. John's wort has been used for years as a folk remedy for depression, but the debate continues on how well it really works, and if it's as safe as it seems.

Ancient healers treated everything from malaria to burns with this herb, but people today use it mainly for depression, anxiety, and sleep disorders. Small studies suggest it helps people with mild depression, perhaps by boosting their brain's serotonin levels the way some antidepressant medications do.

But experts worry that instead of going to their doctor, people will treat themselves for depression. Dr. Richard Nakamura, Acting Director of the National Institute of Mental Health, explains, "Major depression is a serious public health concern. Determining whether an herbal product, such as St. John's wort, can work as a treatment is important."

Look on the bright side. Supplements made from the herb are considered prescription drugs in some European countries. In fact, St. John's wort is the leading treatment for depression in Germany where doctors prescribe it up to 20 times more often than the popular antidepressant Prozac.

A group of researchers recently reviewed over 25 short-term studies on the herb involving thousands of people with depression. In each study, St. John's wort helped relieve mild to moderate depression just as well as traditional tricyclic antidepressants and with fewer side effects.

Have a healthy skepticism. On the other hand, many experts have criticized studies for setting up St. John's wort to look good. To settle the dispute, the National Institutes of Health (NIH) performed a large, well-controlled trial comparing St. John's wort to two other treatments – sertraline (Zoloft), a powerful new antidepressant; and a placebo, fake pills designed to have no effect at all.

Over three hundred people with major depression took part. One group took 900 to 1,500 milligrams (mg) of St. John's wort a day, the second took 50 to 100 mg of sertraline daily, and the third received the placebo. After two months, researchers discovered St. John's wort worked no better than the placebo.

While many studies have shown it could help mild cases of the blues, experts warn not to try treating more serious forms of depression with St. John's wort.

Talk to your doctor if you're feeling down, discuss your options, then arm yourself with these tips for taking the famous herb.

Get the lowdown on side effects. Most studies show St. John's wort has fewer side effects than prescription antidepressants, but the herb can cause dry mouth, dizziness, tiredness, and stomach irritation. It could also make you more sensitive to sunlight, so protect your skin outdoors while taking it.

Watch out for dangerous drug interactions. It may be an herb, but St. John's wort can actually affect the way some prescription drugs work. Dr. Robert Califf of Duke University says, "Remember that a lot of people with other serious illnesses do become depressed and say, 'Well, I'll take a little St. John's wort to perk me up.'

For these people it can be the wrong thing to do without good medical supervision to check these medicines and make sure there's no bad interaction going on."

This perk-me-up becomes a problem when the herb weakens your
other medications. This could
happen with cyclosporine,
digoxin, warfarin, antibiotics, sed-
atives, birth control pills, and certain drugs for depression, heart
disease, cholesterol, seizures, and
some cancers. Interactions like

> **If you already take St. John's wort, tell your doctor during each visit so she knows what medications and dosages to prescribe for other illnesses.**

these make it even more important to see your doctor before
starting St. John's wort.

Be prepared to wait. As with many prescription antidepressants, St. John's wort can take a while to work. Your spirits may
lift in as little as two weeks or as long as eight. Discuss other
treatments with your doctor if you haven't noticed an improvement after two months.

Have a healthy respect for herbs, and they can help you in
return. Just remember – always consult your doctor about natural remedies like this one, and weigh your options carefully.

Other supplements may lift your mood

Dietary supplements by the aisle-full are fighting to edge out
St. John's wort as the new wonder cure for depression.
Before you load up your shopping cart, read on to separate
fact from fiction.

Say hello to "sammy." S-adenosyl-methionine, better known as
SAM-e, is no newcomer to the supplement arena. It has been
prescribed in Europe for both depression and arthritis for over
thirty years.

Your body naturally makes this compound and uses it to build
serotonin, dopamine, and norepinephrine, brain chemicals that
help control your mood. Severely depressed people are often

low in SAM-e, and some experts believe supplements could give your body the boost it needs to lift you out of depression.

The federal government's Agency for Healthcare Research and Quality recently looked at 28 studies on SAM-e and depression. By and large, they discovered that the supplements worked better than placebo – or fake pills – and about as well as prescription drugs in treating depression. And with few side effects.

However, in general, most studies on SAM-e have been short and many used injections rather than the pills sold in stores. These factors could influence test results.

SAM-e may not help everyone, and should never be used to treat bipolar disorder. Experts also warn that SAM-e may improve symptoms of depression but won't necessarily cure it.

Discuss SAM-e with your doctor before taking it so she can advise you and watch your progress. Then check out these tips for getting the most from your supplement.

- SAM-e can break down quickly. Look for supplements sold in sealed, airtight, lightproof containers.

- Buy the enteric-coated tablets to keep them from dissolving before they reach your intestines.

- SAM-e is best taken on an empty stomach, but if it makes you nauseous, try it with food or lower the dosage.

- Vitamin B12 and folate help your body use SAM-e. Look to fish and dairy products for B12, and legumes and fortified cereals for folate.

At one time, half the supplements sold in the United States contained less SAM-e than they actually claimed. For help picking out quality supplements, see *Play it safe when choosing supplements* on page 92 later in this chapter.

Net a better mood. Eicosapentaenoic acid (EPA), one of the omega-3 fatty acids in fish, may work wonders for depression. British researchers gave EPA supplements to 70 depressed people for whom traditional antidepressants had not worked. Twelve weeks later, nearly 70 percent of those receiving 1 gram of EPA daily felt better.

Whole fish and fish oil supplements both contain EPA, but it would be very difficult to get the amounts used in this study just from eating fish. If you're considering fish oil supplements, take 1,000 milligrams (1 gram) of EPA each day since that's the amount that worked best in the study. More isn't necessarily better — larger doses were actually less helpful.

Remember to talk to your doctor before taking fish oil supplements. They're usually made from the fish parts most likely to contain pollutants, and they're naturally rich in vitamins A and D which can be toxic in large doses. In addition, fish oil acts as a natural blood-thinner, so avoid mixing it with aspirin, garlic, ginkgo, or prescription blood-thinning medications.

Get a lift from ginseng. Panax ginseng is one of the "true" ginsengs — not an imitator often passed off for the real thing — and is the most well-researched kind. It's been used to treat fatigue, poor concentration, low energy, and now mental health.

A small group of young adults took 200 milligrams of panax ginseng every day and within four weeks felt more sociable and mentally healthy. But the benefits declined over the next four weeks, which could mean they built up a tolerance to the supplement.

Ginseng is available in several forms, including capsules, teas, soft drinks, dried root, and even chewing gum.

It's too early to tell if ginseng will help depression in the long run, but it may become another weapon in your arsenal. See your doctor before taking ginseng for any ailment.

Play it safe when choosing supplements

Buying dietary supplements may seem as risky as rolling the dice – and too often you're the loser. It's hard to know which products are safe or contain the ingredients they claim. But what if someone you trust could help you pick out the highest quality supplements?

Big-name organizations like U.S. Pharmacopeia are doing just that. They and other organizations now test supplements for quality and safety, then give official-looking seals of approval to those that pass.

Trouble is, not all of these seals make the same promises. Here's your guide to buying what you want and knowing exactly what you're getting.

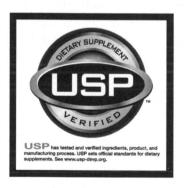

U. S. Pharmacopeia (USP). This non-profit organization has been setting standards for supplements since 1820. In fact, it sets official Food and Drug Administration (FDA) standards for dietary supplements.

Earning a seal of approval from USP through their Dietary Supplement Verification Program isn't easy. Researchers test the supplements in a laboratory and even inspect the manufacturing plants that package them. To get this mark, a supplement must:

- label all of its ingredients.

- actually contain the type and amount of ingredients listed on its label.

- be free of toxins like heavy metals, pesticides, bacteria, or other pollutants.

- have a consistent quality and amount of ingredients in different bottles of the same supplement.

- dissolve completely inside your body.

- label important dosage and warning information.

- be packaged in a safe, clean, controlled environment.

Look for the USP Mark – a green and gold circle containing the letters "USP" – on the supplement's label.

You can get more information about the U.S. Pharmacopeia Dietary Supplement Verification Program on the internet at <www.usp-dsvp.org>.

NSF International. This non-profit organization certifies everything from food and water to dietary supplements. Like USP, NSF tests the products in a lab and inspects the plants where they are packaged. The NSF seal means the supplement:

- clearly labels all of its ingredients.

- contains the ingredients in the amounts listed on its label.

- is free of dangerous contaminants.

- was packaged in a safe, clean environment.

You can spot this seal by looking for the letters "NSF" inside a blue circle with the words "Independently Certified" wrapped around it. Underneath is a box with "Contents Tested" and the organization's Web address.

Go to this Internet site to learn more about NSF's Dietary Supplement Certification Program and which supplements have earned the seal. Or call their Consumer Affairs Office at 1-877-867-3435.

ConsumerLab.com (CL). This private company based in White Plains, N.Y. has made a name for itself independently testing health and nutrition products and publishing the results on their Web site. Now ConsumerLab.com issues its own CL Seal of Approval.

CL tests products in laboratories using industry standards whenever possible, but doesn't inspect the manufacturing plants that package them. What the CL Seal does tell you is that a supplement:

- contains the ingredients and the amounts given on its label.

- is free of harmful contaminants.

- dissolves easily and completely inside your body.

- is the same from one bottle to another.

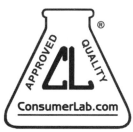

Be Sure It's CL Approved

For dietary supplements, the name of the tested ingredient appears within the seal below the Web address.

You can see a free partial list of the supplements that passed CL's tests on their Web site at <www.consumerlab.com>.

But to see the complete list as well as safety warnings, recalls, and other tips, you have to pay a small fee and subscribe to Consumer-Lab.com as you would to a magazine.

All of these programs are designed to help you separate the good from the bad whenever you buy supplements, but none of these seals guarantees a product is healthy. Never substitute a seal of approval for your doctor's sound advice.

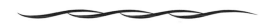

Healthy habits

Depression is not a natural part of aging. It's a curable illness you can overcome with help from loved ones, doctors, and a few savvy survival tips.

Stay healthy. Depression is strongly linked to health issues like chronic illness and physical disability. Seeking treatment for these will help you beat the blues.

Rest up. Sleep is essential in defeating depression, so create good habits. Skip caffeine late in the day, wind down in the evenings, and stick to a regular bedtime.

Get physical. A long walk could put a smile on your face. Exercise lowers stress, increases energy, and takes your mind off your problems.

Lean on loved ones. Build a support group of friends and family and call on them when you're feeling down. They'll help you see the bright side and battle the low times.

Focus on short-term goals. Get out of bed, brush your teeth, walk the dog – meeting small goals can keep you motivated during dark times.

CHAPTER 11 *Diabetes*

What is diabetes? You develop diabetes when your body can't properly produce or use insulin. This hormone helps your cells transform food into energy for everyday life. The two main kinds of diabetes are Type 1 (insulin-dependent) and Type 2 (noninsulin-dependent diabetes mellitus).

Who gets it? Seniors, blacks, Latinos, Native Americans, and Asians have an increased risk. You're more at risk, too, if it's in your family or you're overweight.

What are the symptoms?

- frequent urination
- excessive thirst or increased appetite
- unexplained weight loss
- blurry vision

Check out this new eating plan

Move over low-fat, high-carbohydrate diet. There's a new way to eat if you're diabetic. Experts from the American Diabetes Association (ADA) came up with a delicious eating plan that centers around monounsaturated fatty acids (MUFAs), the good kind of fat.

"We found that a diet rich in monounsaturated fatty acids led to improvement in HDL (high-density lipoprotein) cholesterol, triglycerides and, most importantly, diabetes control," announces Dr. Abhimanyu Garg, a member of the ADA's expert panel.

That means MUFAs could help manage your insulin and blood sugar levels and fight diabetes-related heart disease.

Monounsaturated fats. As the rising star in diabetes control, MUFAs make up a big part of the new ADA eating plan. Along with carbohydrates, they should make up 60 to 70 percent of your daily calories. You can find these good fats in avocados, peanut butter, peanuts, almonds, cashews, pecans, and olive, canola, and peanut oils.

Polyunsaturated fats. These other "good" fats are also beneficial in moderate amounts – up to 10 percent of your calories. For heart-healthy omega-3 PUFAs, eat two servings a week of salmon, halibut, herring, mackerel, or other fatty fish. Flaxseed, flaxseed oil, canola oil, and walnuts are also excellent sources. For omega-6, another type of PUFA, try spreads and oils made from corn, sunflower, and safflower.

Carbohydrates. "As far as the carbohydrate-containing foods are concerned," Garg says, "it's best to use unrefined carbohydrates instead of sucrose. If you get your carbohydrates from fruits, vegetables, and grains, then there are other beneficial substances that are not included in a package of sugar."

Garg is talking about vitamins, minerals, and antioxidants – not to mention fiber. Fiber is the one substance that may cleanse your system and help it win the battle against diabetes, heart disease, stroke, impotence, and cancer. In one study, a very high-fiber diet, about 50 grams, lowered blood sugar levels by 10 percent. Fruits, vegetables, and whole-grain breads and cereals are great sources of fiber.

The new ADA guidelines permit a sweet treat now and then. Just make sure to count it in your daily carbohydrate ratio. Ultimately, it's more important to watch how many carbs you eat – not what kind they are.

Protein. Another 15 to 20 percent of your daily calories in the ADA eating plan should be protein. Any more than this – like the amount in high-protein diets – could cause long-term health problems, such as high cholesterol. The wrong kind of protein can cause health problems, too. Some sources are loaded with saturated fat and cholesterol. The ADA guidelines suggest limiting your intake of saturated fats, found in meat, egg yolks, whole milk, butter, and cheese, to less than 10 percent of your daily calories.

Saturated fat reverses many of the benefits of MUFAs. Eating too much "bad" fat can raise your blood pressure and your LDL cholesterol. Saturated fat can even worsen your insulin resistance, making it harder to control your blood sugar. You should also keep your dietary cholesterol to less than 300 milligrams (mg) a day. To give you an idea how much cholesterol that is, a cup of whole milk contains 35 mg, a croissant has about 50 mg, a half-cup serving of Fettucine alfredo has 60 mg, and a batter-dipped, fried chicken breast has a whopping 238 mg of cholesterol.

> **Here's a general guideline — the more saturated a fat is, the more solid it is at room temperature.**

To limit saturated fat and cholesterol, swap low-fat dairy products for their fatty counterparts. Replace butter, lard, and margarine with spreads and oils made from corn, sunflower, and safflower oils. Then eat fish, legumes, bulgur, and rice for your protein instead of meat.

When it comes to options, this new eating plan gives you plenty. "Now diabetics can choose a diet rich in carbohydrates," says Garg, "or a diet rich in monounsaturated fats." It's up to you and your doctor to decide the best way to control your diabetes, prevent heart disease, maintain a healthy weight, and – best of all – please your taste buds.

Try natural healers from your kitchen

Your grandfather might have had a hand in your diabetes, according to a curious new study from Europe. His eating habits as a child could have raised your risk of dying from diabetes.

Although this is intriguing news, it doesn't help you now if you suffer from diabetes. The most important thing you can do today is make each calorie count. Instead of junk food, fit these tasty foods into your eating plan. They'll add flavor and diversity to your menu. But more importantly, they are natural healing alternatives for diabetes that don't require drugs, doctors, or lab tests.

Say 'nuts' to diabetes. Researchers with the Nurses' Health Study recently looked at the relationship between nuts and diabetes risk, and they liked what they saw. Women in the study who ate an ounce of nuts — about a handful — at least five times a week had a 27-percent less chance of developing Type 2 diabetes, compared with women who almost never ate them.

"We were not really surprised by our findings," announces Rui Jiang, one of the study's authors. "Nuts contain lots of fat, but most fats in nuts are mono- and polyunsaturated fats, which are good for insulin sensitivity and serum cholesterol. Nuts are also rich in antioxidant vitamins, minerals, plant protein, and dietary fiber."

Jiang suggests adding these nutrient powerhouses to your diet. "To avoid increase in caloric intake," she advises, "people should not simply add nuts on the top of the diet. Instead, people should substitute nuts for less-healthy foods such as refined carbohydrates, like white bread and red meats."

Roast a chicken. Eating chicken seems to treat microalbuminuria, a complication that affects one out of five diabetics and can lead to heart and kidney problems.

Normally, diabetics at risk for microalbuminuria go on a strict low-protein diet or take expensive drugs. Choosing chicken as a source of protein instead of red meat is a tastier and effective alternative. The chicken's low saturated fat content and its polyunsaturated fat may explain its benefits.

Fill your mug with coffee. Java junkies, rejoice. A recent European study found that drinking seven or more cups of coffee a day may cut your risk of Type 2 diabetes in half. This finding was surprising since caffeine has been shown to decrease insulin sensitivity in another study.

This new research followed more than 17,000 people for 13 years. During that time, the researchers discovered coffee contains beneficial compounds, too. But don't overdo it. Drinking too much coffee could have adverse effects. Talk with your doctor about what this study means for you.

Enjoy a glass of low-fat milk. Fortified milk is chock-full of nutrients, but the most important one for diabetics may be vitamin A. Research suggests vitamin A may help insulin work more effectively. Liver is also one of the vitamin's top natural sources.

Or you could turn to brightly colored fruits and vegetables, like sweet potatoes, carrots, spinach, and cantaloupe. They are high in beta carotene, and your body uses beta carotene to make vitamin A.

Send in the salmon. This fatty, cold-water fish is a top source of omega-3 fatty acids. Besides all their other health benefits, these good fats may also improve your insulin sensitivity. That's one more reason to eat two servings a week of salmon, halibut, herring, mackerel, or other cold-water fish.

> Just one-fourth to one teaspoon of cinnamon every day can help your fat cells recognize and respond to insulin better. Sprinkle some on your favorite foods.

Give olive oil a chance. Not only does this oil give you a dose of monounsaturated fatty acids, it's full of vitamin E, too. This powerful antioxidant vitamin could protect you from free radical damage, and it might even help prevent diabetes.

Ginseng berry offers hope

The ginseng root usually gets all the attention in the herbal world, but now the ginseng berry is stealing the show as a possible diabetes treatment.

"We were stunned by how different the berry is from the root and by how effective it is in correcting the multiple metabolic abnormalities associated with diabetes," testifies Dr. Chun-Su Yuan, assistant professor at the University of Chicago.

Yuan's research team recently tested an extract of the berry. They discovered it could balance blood sugar and improve insulin sensitivity. Moreover, it appeared to cut cholesterol levels and lower weight.

The secret to these outstanding results may be a compound called ginsenoside Re. Ginseng berries are loaded with it, while the roots aren't.

Don't rush to buy bushels of these wonder berries. The study used mice, so more work needs to be done to see if the ginseng berry works for people.

Still, Yuan claims, "Since this berry contains agents that are effective against both obesity and diabetes, the ginseng fruit has enormous promise as a source of new drugs."

Fruits and veggies to the rescue

Vegetables and fruits should always make up a big part of your diet, but if you're diabetic, they're even more important. And here's why – they contain vitamins and minerals that attack diabetes head on.

Gain ground with grapes. A natural grape compound called pterostilbene could lower blood sugar, fight diabetes, and even take on cancer. Dr. Agnes M. Rimando, a chemist with the U.S. Department of Agriculture who researches this odd-sounding substance says, "My study is saying that there's another compound in grapes with equal cancer-fighting power as resveratrol, but which has antidiabetic properties as well."

Rimando and other scientists have only done test-tube and animal studies, so more research on pterostilbene needs to be done. Still, eating grapes is healthy no matter how you look at it. Pick dark-skinned varieties over light ones. They contain more pterostilbene.

> **Squirt some lemon juice on your meals just before you eat. You'll get a jolt of vitamin C. Plus, the acidity could help slow your digestion and steady your blood sugar.**

Snack on figs. The American Diabetes Association doesn't recommend figs for nothing. They're a high-fiber snack. Just five figs have 9 grams of fiber. Fiber slows down the conversion of carbohydrates into sugar. And foods high in fiber tend to cause your body to produce less insulin. Besides, figs are delicious and make a super substitute for candy or cookies.

Steam some broccoli. Like nuts, broccoli is packed with a bounty of treasures, such as magnesium. If you take insulin for your diabetes, you're at risk for a magnesium deficiency, which could increase your chances of complications. So feast on raw or lightly cooked broccoli crowns, as well as other sources of magnesium, like beans, shellfish, and whole grains.

Get friendly with lima beans. You're likely to be low in zinc if you're diabetic, and that's dangerous for your eyes. A deficiency of this mineral can lead to damage of your retina and eventually blindness. Consider adding top sources like lima beans, meat, shellfish, and whole grains to your diet.

Slice up sweet red peppers. The boatload of vitamin C in these delicious vegetables can help control your blood sugar level and improve insulin sensitivity. Plus, vitamin C is an antioxidant, so it protects you from heart disease. Other sources include citrus fruits, strawberries, broccoli, and brussels sprouts.

Shield yourself with garlic and onions. Last but not least, these flavor powerhouses can come to your aid. Experts say sulfur-containing compounds in the bulbs could help lower your blood sugar levels.

Quick tips to boost low blood sugar

Sudden grouchiness, hunger, or tiredness might not just be a passing mood. If you're diabetic, it could be a sign of hypoglycemia or low blood sugar.

Hypoglycemia occurs when your blood sugar dips too low. Other symptoms include weakness, confusion, sweating, headache, shakiness, or even coma and seizures.

If you experience any of these symptoms, take action quickly by following these steps to recovery from the National Institutes of Health.

Check your blood sugar level. A reading of 70 or lower means you are hypoglycemic. To raise your blood sugar back to a safe level, try one of these fast-acting remedies:

- half a cup of fruit juice or regular (not diet) soda
- a piece of fruit or small box of raisins
- five or six pieces of hard candy
- one to two teaspoons of sugar or honey
- two to three store-bought glucose tablets

Carry one of these quick fixes with you at all times. If you take insulin, keep a glucagon kit with you, too. It can quickly raise your blood glucose level.

Wait 15 minutes. Check your blood sugar again to make sure it's no longer too low.

Make sure a meal is on the horizon. Once your blood sugar level is stable, plan to eat a meal within the next hour. If you can't, snack on one of the following:

- crackers, peanut butter, or cheese crackers
- half a sandwich
- a serving of milk or yogurt

Prevent future incidents. Don't gamble with your blood sugar level. Managing it is a matter of discipline and good sense. So eat regular meals and avoid alcohol. Take your medication as prescribed. Check your blood sugar often. And last but not least, exercise with care.

Cooking trick might tame heart villain

It's not what you cook that's important. It's how you cook it. Chemicals called advanced glycation end products (AGEs) are the reason.

These components form naturally when foods containing sugars, fats, and proteins are cooked at high temperatures for a long time.

Although scientists have known about AGEs for a while, they only recently discovered the danger to diabetics. In fact, according to the latest research from New York's Mount Sinai School of Medicine, AGEs could be a major reason why diabetics are at high risk for heart disease.

The researchers suspect AGEs cause a diabetic's immune system to overreact, which could eventually damage blood vessels. But there's good news.

You can control the amount of AGEs you consume. Follow these tips to lower the number of AGEs in your food.

- **Limit animal foods.** Out of more than 200 foods tested for AGEs, animal foods cooked at high temperatures topped the list, especially those high in fat and protein like meat, cheese, and egg yolks.

- **Change the way you cook.** High-humidity cooking methods, like boiling and steaming, could produce less AGEs in your food. Quick cooking at low heat, like stir frying, is another healthy option. Just remember – baking, grilling, and broiling could be harmful to your blood vessels.

Though the Mount Sinai research is in its early stages, it can't hurt to follow these recommendations now. They could also protect you from kidney disease and other complications.

Digesting the Glycemic Index controversy

You probably know about the controversy brewing around the Glycemic Index (GI). But do you know what it means for you?

The Pros. According to a Harvard study, you can control your blood sugar by eating a diet of low-GI carbohydrates. These are carbohydrates your body breaks down into glucose at a steady pace. High-GI foods, on the other hand, are absorbed quickly and send your blood sugar skyrocketing.

The Cons. It's not that easy to predict what will happen to your blood sugar when you eat a certain food, contend GI critics. The food's ripeness, its preparation, and its total nutrient content affect the GI. Your metabolism does, too. That's why the American Diabetic Association (ADA) suggests you monitor how many – not what kind of – carbohydrates you eat.

The Solution. There is common ground between the ADA and the Harvard researchers. They both recommend eating more complex carbohydrates like whole grains. That's healthy advice any way you look at it.

Another option is the Glycemic Load (GL), which could be an easier, more accurate way to figure a food's effect on your blood sugar. Read more about it in *Rank your carbs to get thin* on page 324.

Healthy habits

An exciting new treatment for Type 2 diabetes is on the horizon. It's a hormone called GLP-1 that might help you control your blood sugar and lose weight. Unfortunately, GLP-1 is still in the experimental stage. In the meantime, control your diabetes with these proven tips.

- Ask your doctor how many meals and snacks you should eat and how often to check your blood sugar.
- Eat about the same time every day, and don't skip meals and snacks. Measure your food to be sure you are eating the same amount.
- Take medication at the same time every day.
- Ask your doctor to help you design an exercise program. Then exercise around the same time each day. This amazing remedy could help you lose weight, reduce stress, and even treat your diabetes.
- Wear comfortable shoes. Keep your feet clean and dry. Inspect them regularly for redness or sores, especially after exercise. Report problems to your doctor.
- Lose weight if you're overweight. Even dropping 10 to 20 pounds helps.

CHAPTER 12 *Forgetfulness*

What is forgetfulness? It's an ongoing failure to remember new information and recent events.

Who gets it? This condition is generally associated with getting older, but seniors are aging better when it comes to memory. Only about 4 percent of people over 70 have serious memory problems. Women over 85 typically have a better memory than men of the same age.

What are the symptoms?

- difficulty recalling names and other familiar information
- frequent problems finding misplaced objects
- confusion

Turn back the clock with fruits and veggies

"It's not the '60s. Beware of free radicals," advises Dr. Gary Small in his book, *The Memory Bible*. He isn't talking about hippies, but if you have trouble remembering back to those flower-power days, listen up.

Free radicals, Small points out, are oxidants that can do serious harm to your brain cells. Fortunately, vitamins C and E can help combat this damage. "Recent studies," says Small, "show that people with low blood levels of these antioxidant vitamins have poorer memory abilities."

Scientists at Tufts University created a scale to rate the antioxidant power of foods. They place these among the most potent.

- **Blueberries, blackberries, strawberries, and raspberries.** Enjoy these delicious and nutritious morsels on cereals, in salads, or by themselves as a sweet treat.

- **Prunes and raisins.** These dried fruits are high in calories, so alternate them with fresh ones like red grapes, oranges, plums, and cherries.

- **Colorful veggies.** Green spinach, broccoli, and avocado; red bell peppers and beets; yellow corn; and purple eggplant can brighten your brain with antioxidants.

> Boron is an amazing mineral that prevents "mental meltdown." It's not considered "essential," but we know it affects everything from hand-eye coordination to long- and short-term memory.

Antioxidant vitamins aren't the only ones you need to protect your memory. "Almost any vitamin deficiency," Small says, "will affect brain fitness and should be avoided." In fact, a B-vitamin deficiency is one of the first things he tests for when a patient complains of forgetfulness.

Include fish, lean meats, cereals, and leafy greens in your diet to be sure you are getting all the important B vitamins. For the brain-boosting minerals zinc, iron, and boron, add nuts, whole grains, and dried beans.

Rev up your 'recall' with a low-fat diet

The kind of gas you put in your car can determine how well your engine runs. It's no surprise that your brain operates better on the right kind of fuel, too. While a high-fat diet can make your brain sluggish, a low-fat diet keeps it operating smoothly.

"Our brain needs glucose — essentially energy — in order to function," says researcher Dr. Carol Greenwood of the Baycrest Centre for Geriatric Care and the University of Toronto. But saturated fatty acids can keep your brain from using glucose effectively. "It's like clogging the brain and starving it of energy," she says.

Greenwood and fellow researcher Dr. Gordon Winocur studied the effects of a high-fat diet on memory in rats. They found those who ate a lot of fat were slower to learn simple tasks and remember how to perform them when compared with the rats that ate a low-fat diet.

Although after treatment with glucose their memories improved, Winocur points out that increasing glucose isn't a substitute for a healthy diet.

"We should not fool ourselves," he says, "into thinking that glucose from a glass of orange juice is all we need to protect our brains from clogging up from a high-fat diet."

Greenwood agrees. "The one message I hope people take away from this study," she says, "is that modifying the diet and lowering fat intake is good for your brain function."

> Sip a cup of coffee. Both caffeine and a bit of sugar will stave off memory loss. But avoid the artificial sweetener aspartame. It could make your forgetfulness worse.

The fats used in the study were beef tallow and soybean oil. The results might be different using moderate amounts of olive oil – a good fat that buffers the brain against memory loss – or fish oil, with brain-healthy omega-3 fatty acids.

To keep your memory sharp from start to finish, drop the high-fat breakfast of bacon, eggs, and buttered toast. Instead have a bowl of oatmeal and a banana. These carbohydrates provide fast energy to your noggin. And watch the fats in other meals as well. Your brain, your heart, and your waistline will thank you.

Grow in wisdom with herbs

Time spent strolling or working in your garden reduces stress. And that's always good for your brain. But for better circulation, more energy, and greater concentration – which also help improve your mental performance – try these savory garden herbs.

> Yellow mustard has more antioxidants than the darker Dijon variety. That's due to the curcumin in the turmeric, the spice that gives mustard its bright yellow color.

Garlic. This powerful herb fights clogged arteries and helps get more blood to your brain for clearer thinking.

Garlic bread is one popular way to add this powerful protector to your diet. Mix crushed garlic, olive oil, and dried oregano together. Spread it between slices of French bread, wrap it in foil, and pop it in the oven until warm. You can also add generous amounts of garlic to soups, casseroles, and spaghetti sauce.

Rosemary. This savory herb, rich in antioxidants, is said to help improve concentration and long-term memory. Even the scent can make you more alert. Add it to stews and meat dishes for mouth-watering flavor and clearer thinking.

Chamomile. A soothing cup of chamomile tea helps reduce anxiety. What's more, the scent of this herb also helps calm your nerves and cheer up your sluggish brain.

Lavender. It's hard to focus when you are stressed, but you'll bounce back – bright and energetic – after a relaxing walk beside a fragrant bed of lavender. And for better circulation, soak your feet in a warm bath scented with lavender oil.

Ginseng. This ancient herb helps boost energy and concentration, but it grows slowly in your garden. And since most of the studies that show the benefits used Asian plants, it's probably best to buy it from a health food store instead of trying to grow your own.

5 tips for a sharper memory

- Make gestures with your hands while you talk.
- Use all your senses. Recall the color and scent of a flower, for example, to remember its name.
- Sing your "to do" or grocery list to a favorite tune.
- Retrace your steps – physically or mentally – to find a misplaced item.
- Write down what you do remember about a topic in order to recall details you have forgotten.

Chew on this to recharge your memory

Could chewing gum help your memory? Scientists at Northumbria University in England asked that question recently after noticing that lab rats unable to chew also had poor memories.

To find out how chewing affects humans, the researchers conducted a study in which they divided people into three groups. A third of the participants chewed gum, another third pretended to chew but had nothing in their mouths, and the remaining group neither chewed nor pretended to chew. After 30 minutes, they were all given memory tests.

"We found a very clear pattern of improved memory when gum was chewed," says Dr. Andrew Scholey. In fact, the gum chewers remembered an impressive 35 percent more than the other two groups.

The real gum chewers had a faster heart rate by five to six beats per minute than the others. Dr. Scholey believes that might – at least in part – explain the results. "The increase in heart rate leads to an increase in blood flow and therefore delivers more oxygen and glucose to the brain," he says.

Another possible explanation is that chewing stimulates the production of insulin, which may affect the hippocampus, the area of the brain responsible for memory. In any case, Dr. Scholey thinks it's the chewing action itself, not something in the gum, that improves the brain's performance.

If that's true, chewing your food more thoroughly might be another way to help your brain – and you'll improve your digestion, too.

Soy linked to faster brain aging

Go slow on soy foods – tofu, miso, veggie burgers, and soy dogs – if you want to hold on to your memory. In light of all the publicity about the health benefits of soy, does this suggestion surprise you?

"You should not be comforted by the multitude of voices praising soy foods," says Dr. Lon White, who continues to be concerned about the connection between soy and forgetfulness he discovered over three years ago.

At that time, White and his fellow researchers at the Pacific Health Research Institute in Hawaii examined the eating patterns of more than 8,000 Japanese-American men over a period of 30 years.

They found that those who ate two or more servings of tofu a week were far more likely to have memory problems as they got older than those who ate little or no tofu. And the more tofu they ate, the greater their memory and learning difficulties.

Just because a food comes from plants, White points out, doesn't mean it's necessarily healthy. What bothers him is that isoflavones, the molecules that supposedly give soy its health benefits, act more like drugs than nutrients and carry the risk of harmful side effects.

White doesn't suggest you avoid soy altogether, but he does recommend keeping to moderate amounts. Although many foods contain some soy, he says people tend to get the most isoflavones from eating tofu.

The typical Asian diet includes one to three servings of tofu per week. Eating more than that, White says, "may be associated with an accumulating risk for ill health, including more rapid brain aging."

Hang out with friends for richer memories

Remember the days when you got into trouble for going out with your friends when you should have been studying? Maybe that wasn't such a bad idea after all. In fact, yakking with your friends – believe it or not – could help preserve your brain.

"As the population ages, interest has been growing about how to maintain healthy brains and minds," says Oscar Ybarra. As a research psychologist at the University of Michigan, he investigates ways to do just that.

In a study of 3,617 Americans between ages 24 and 96, Ybarra discovered a strong connection between being socially active and having a sharp working memory. Those who spent the most time involved in activities with others – no matter what their age – scored the highest on memory tests. They showed less mental decline on other tests, as well.

"Most advice for preserving and enhancing mental function emphasizes intellectual activities such as reading, doing cross-word puzzles, and learning how to use a computer," says Dr.

Ybarra. "But my research suggests that just getting together and chatting with friends and family may also be effective."

Ybarra says these findings also cut across cultural lines. In a different study, for example, he discovered that those people living in the Middle East who were most actively involved with family and friends were better at remembering, making decisions, and succeeding at other mental tasks.

In light of Ybarra's research, this might be a good time to put down your newspaper, call a few good friend, and make a date to get together for some schmoozing.

Healthy habits

Remember these healthy ways to keep your memory in tip-top shape:

- Don't skip meals.
- Exercise regularly.
- Wear warm clothing to avoid hypothermia.
- Keep learning.
- Stay in close contact with loved ones.
- Listen to music to reduce stress.
- Get plenty of sleep
- Don't smoke.
- Limit alcohol.

CHAPTER 13 *Gallstones*

What are gallstones? They are a solid mass of choles-terol that form in the gallbladder or bile ducts. They cause pain when they get too big or block bile ducts that connect the gallbladder and liver or small intestine.

Who gets them? One in 10 Americans get gallstones, especially older people. Before age 60, women get them more than men. After age 60, the risk is equal. Being over-weight or having recently lost a lot of weight; taking choles-terol-lowering drugs; having diabetes; and a family history of gallstones all increase the risk. The genetic odds are greater for Native Americans and Hispanics.

What are the symptoms? Most gallstones produce no symptoms, but when they do, they most likely are pain; chills and fever; yellow or jaundiced skin and whites of eyes; and pale, clay-colored stools.

An orange a day keeps gallstones at bay

A large orange every day might be all it takes to prevent painful gallstones if you have a low level of vitamin C, or ascorbic acid, in your bloodstream.

"Although a few previous studies have shown a relationship between vitamin C and gallbladder disease," says Dr. Joel Simon of the San Francisco Veterans Affairs Medical Center, "the size of our study and the collection of data on undetected gallstones strengthens the hypothesis that vitamin C levels may be an important risk factor for gallstone formation, at least among women."

In this study of more than 13,000 people, the females who increased the vitamin C in their blood by .05 milligrams per

---

deciliter – which is equal to about one large orange a day – reduced their risk of painful gallbladder disease by 13 percent.

While the results weren't as strong for men, Simon believes vitamin C is important for them, too. He thinks the outcome of the study could be due to a biological difference in men and women.

But it's possible the outcome may have been affected by the fact that men don't get gallbladder disease as often as women.

Simon's advice is simple, "Eat your fruits and vegetables." Choose citrus fruits, dark leafy greens, and other bright-colored fruits and vegetables. You'll not only get lots of vitamin C and other nutrients, you'll get fiber, which is also necessary for a healthy gallbladder.

As important as it is to say yes to fruits and vegetables, it's equally important to say no to these foods:

Fatty cuts of meat and full-fat dairy products. Eating a lot of saturated fat in foods like these increases your risk of developing gallstones. That's because they can raise your cholesterol, an ingredient of most gallstones.

Pastries, desserts, and sweet beverages. Foods high in refined sugars also increase your chances of getting gallstones, probably because they increase insulin and, in turn, cholesterol.

Chili peppers. A study in Chile found that poor people who eat lots of hot chili peppers are more likely to get gallbladder cancer. The people in the study also ate fewer fresh fruits. So, if you like chilli peppers, eat lots of fresh oranges, apples, and bananas, too.

Pickles, cabbage, and fried foods. Steer clear of these foods if you already have gallbladder problems, since foods like these may cause you pain.

Healthy habits

Use these tips to enjoy a healthy, gallstone-free life.

- Eat smaller meals.
- Maintain a healthy weight.
- Avoid very low-calorie and yo-yo (losing and gaining weight again and again) diets.
- Exercise often.
- Think twice about hormone replacement therapy. It may increase your risk of gallstones.

Coffee beans blast gallstones

Do you wonder if drinking caffeinated coffee every day is good for you? As far as your gallbladder is concerned, the answer is yes.

The Harvard Nurses' Health study, which followed 80,898 women for 20 years, found that those drinking four cups of coffee a day had gallbladder surgery about 25 percent less often than those who didn't drink coffee. And the more coffee they drank – at least up through five cups – the more it seemed to protect their gallbladders.

Keep in mind drinking that much coffee isn't a good idea for everybody. It may increase your risk of rheumatoid arthritis.

"Women should not start drinking coffee just to prevent gallstone disease," advises lead researcher Dr. Michael F. Leitzmann. "However, if a woman already happens to be a coffee drinker, our study suggests that it is okay for her to continue drinking coffee in terms of her risk of gallstone disease."

> **Eat breakfast. This encourages your bladder to contract and flush out bile and any stones that may be forming after overnight fasting.**

Decaffeinated coffee drinkers didn't fare so well in the study, but researchers say it's still not clear caffeine, rather than something else in coffee, makes the difference. Leitzmann, however, says there's some evidence caffeine causes the gallbladder to contract, which might keep gallstones from forming. Although only women were included in this study, earlier studies have shown similar results for men as well.

CHAPTER 14

Gout

What is gout? Gout is a type of arthritis caused from a buildup of uric acid in your body. Either you make too much of this natural substance or your kidneys can't flush it out. It crystallizes in your joints, causing pain and inflammation. If not treated, gout attacks can become chronic, crippling your joints and limiting movement.

Who gets it? Gout tends to run in families, and men seem more likely to develop it than women. High blood pressure, obesity, alcohol abuse, and insulin resistance all raise your risk for gout.

What are the symptoms?

- sharp, excruciating joint pain, often in the big toe
- swollen, tender, warm, or red joint(s)
- mild fever

Amazing new diet may end gout

Suffering from gout used to mean a strict diet that cut out many popular foods. But new research is challenging the old notions of what's good and bad for this type of arthritis.

Throw out the old. Two things are certain – being overweight and having high levels of uric acid in your blood send your risk for gout through the roof. So traditional treatments have focused on losing those extra pounds and cutting out foods high in purines, a protein that breaks down into uric acid inside your body.

You'd have to skip many of your favorite foods to avoid purines, most meat, seafood, alcohol, and many plant foods such as spinach and beans are bursting with them. On top of that, you'd need to watch your weight. Most people can't stick to a strict regimen like this for very long.

Welcome the new. Evidence now shows that cutting out purine-rich foods has little effect on uric acid. Many experts think it's time to change the game plan.

Enter the modern gout diet. Scientists originally created it for people who were insulin resistant (IR), a condition linked to diabetes, high blood pressure, and heart disease. Like gout, IR is also marked by high uric acid levels, leading researchers to believe too much uric acid could be a warning sign of other, more serious health problems.

Thirteen men with gouty arthritis tried the new diet for four months. They lost an average of 17 pounds, dropped their uric acid levels by almost 20 percent, had two-thirds fewer flare-ups, and even lowered their cholesterol. Best of all, most of them managed to stay on the diet and maintain these benefits for over a year.

Don't try to control your weight through crash diets or fasting. These actually raise your body's uric acid levels and could bring on a gout attack.

The new plan is simple. Eat no more than 1600 calories a day. Get 30 percent of those (480 calories) from protein, 30 percent from fat, and 40 percent (640 calories) from carbohydrates. There's no limit on purine-rich foods, but weight loss is still a major goal.

Boosting your proteins, fats, and carbs, though, doesn't mean you can eat a T-bone steak every night, load up on fatty french fries, or munch all the potato chips you want. The focus is on eating healthier sources of these nutrients. Here are a few insider tips to make the most of this diet.

- **Cut back on calories.** Divide those 1600 calories among three to five small meals throughout the day, rather than two or three large ones.

- **Swap out the fats.** Cut back on saturated fats found in foods like dairy products, and load up instead on heart-healthy unsaturated fats in fish, poultry, nuts, peanut butter, avocados, and olive and canola oils.

- **Be smart about carbohydrates.** Choose the complex sugars in fruits and vegetables rather than the refined sugars in candy, chips, and sodas.

- **Eat more fish.** The men in this study ate at least four servings of fish each week including salmon, haddock, mackerel, and trout – terrific sources of protein and healthy polyunsaturated fatty acids.

> **If your doctor tells you to avoid high-purine foods, you'll have to skip the fish, a rich source.**

Discuss this eating plan with your doctor if you think it could work for you. While diet can make a difference, many medications can also help ease your gout pain and prevent future flare-ups. Go over your choices before trying to treat yourself.

Beware of drugs that trigger gout

When it comes to gout, the danger isn't all in what you eat. Certain drugs can also set you up for painful attacks.

Aspirin. Even as little as 75 milligrams (mg) of aspirin can affect how well your kidneys flush out uric acid, a serious problem for gout sufferers. While heart-saving daily doses of baby aspirin are still generally considered safe, experts warn against taking large doses such as 1,000 to 2,000 mg if you have gout.

Water pills. Doctors often prescribe these drugs, known as thiazide diuretics, for high blood pressure, but they've been linked to gout in older women with kidney problems.

Allopurinol. This medication is actually used to treat gout, but it can trigger flare-ups when you first begin taking it. It is top- notch at preventing future attacks, so make sure you stick with it for the full benefits.

Discuss these risks with your doctor, and never take yourself off any medications without her supervision.

Rout gout with smart menu choices

Just three dried cherries a day could end your gout pain. It may sound like a miracle, but this delicious, vitamin-packed fruit is proven to relieve arthritis pain even better than aspirin, ibuprofen and other drugs – with no stomach upset or other side effects.

The secret lies in anthocyanins. These natural compounds not only give cherries their luscious red color – they also stop your body from making prostaglandins, the hormone-like substances that cause pain and inflammation.

In lab studies, anthocyanins have proven to be about ten times more effective than aspirin at relieving joint pain and swelling. That's a huge plus, because even small amounts of aspirin can worsen gout.

With this fruit in hand, you may not even need to take pain pills. Instead, you can let cherries ease the ache of this arthritis. Experts recommend munching cherries every day during a gout attack. Pop a few dried ones in your mouth, or eat a bowl full of fresh ones instead. About three dried cherries pack the same punch as 20 fresh ones.

These sweet fruits aren't the only gout-busting foods. Read on to discover more ways of taking the sting out of this disease.

Wash it away with water. If you suffer from gout and drink water only when you're thirsty, you may not be drinking enough. Water cushions achy joints, and is crucial in flushing uric acid out of your body.

If you have gout, you need plenty of this fluid to keep your body's machinery running in tip-top condition. Make it your main beverage. Drink it in place of sugary sodas, and spice it up with a twist of lemon or lime. You can also carry small bottles of water with you wherever you go, and sip them throughout the day.

Not everyone needs eight glasses of water a day, but according to the Johns Hopkins Medical Institutions, you should drink at least enough to produce two liters of urine a day.

Ask your doctor how much is best for you, then go after gout just by drinking the right amount.

Mooove over, arthritis. Ditching gout could be as easy as eating more dairy products. Getting 30 grams or more of dairy protein each day helped people put the lid on their levels of uric acid in a recent Canadian study.

A single serving of yogurt with its 12 grams of protein puts you well on your way to filling that quota. Add another 8 grams from a cup of milk, and you'll soon be saying goodbye to gout.

Give three cheers for coffee. Natural chemicals in this morning motivator may also lower the uric acid in your blood. Both instant and brewed coffee seem to have an anti-gout effect. Surprisingly, green tea did not.

It's too early to tell just how effective coffee is, but since it's low in purines — a kind of protein that breaks down into uric acid — your daily cup of java probably won't hurt. Talk to your doctor, though, before drinking more coffee than usual to treat your gout.

You may have to take medication to control active cases of gout, but eating right can help you get back on your feet and kick this painful illness.

Healthy habits

Soothe the ache with ice. Putting an ice pack on sore joints may ease the pain during flare-ups. Don't have an ice pack handy? Use a bag of frozen peas instead.

Take it easy. Stay in bed both during a gout attack and for at least 24 hours after the pain passes. Moving around too soon can aggravate the inflamed joint and trigger another gout attack.

Steer clear of alcohol. Drinking alcohol puts you at greater risk for developing gout and can make attacks more severe.

Get moving once you're better. Obesity and high blood pressure are two big risk factors for gout. In addition to changing your diet, work with your doctor on a mild exercise program that can put the squeeze on these serious health problems.

CHAPTER 15

Headache

What is a headache? There are three main types of head-aches – tension headaches, migraines, and cluster head-aches. Headaches can be caused by stress, exhaustion, repressed anger, muscle contractions, and expanding or contracting blood vessels in and around your brain.

Who gets it? Almost everyone has experienced a tension headache. Women are much more likely to get migraines, while men are more prone to cluster headaches.

What are the symptoms? Dull, sharp, or throbbing pain, tightness, and pressure in your forehead, temples, or the back of your head.

Sometimes a headache can be a symptom of a more serious medical problem, such as an infection or tumor. See your doctor if you have frequent and severe headaches.

Cook up some migraine relief

If you suddenly see lights, don't worry – it's not a UFO. It's probably an aura, colored spots that flash before your eyes when a migraine is on its way.

Migraines affect up to 18 percent of women and 6 percent of men. The pounding pain, which often sends you straight to bed, can also make you nauseous, irritable, and overly sensitive to light and sound.

Though some foods can trigger a migraine, plenty of others help you heal. This delicious sample meal contains several powerful migraine busters.

- Fillet of salmon seasoned with ginger

- Sauteed spinach and mushrooms

- A glass of fortified milk

Salmon. This fish is loaded with omega-3 fatty acids, which help control inflammation. These helpful fats can cut some migraines off before they even start. In a study held in Cincinnati, about 60 percent of the participants had fewer and less severe migraines after taking fish oil supplements for six weeks.

Though fish oil capsules are an easy way to get your omega-3, an even better way is from natural sources. Look for omega-3 in cold-water fish like salmon, tuna, mackerel, and sardines. It's also found in flaxseed and wheat germ.

Ginger. If you want milder and less frequent migraines, this is the rhizome for you. A Danish woman suffering from frequent migraines drank a mixture of powdered ginger and plain water during an attack and noticed her headache was less severe. She started eating raw ginger regularly and had fewer migraines.

Ginger, often taken to ease motion sickness, may also calm the nausea that frequently accompanies migraines.

To reap the benefits of ginger, you have to eat 2 to 4 grams a day – a relatively large amount. You can either eat the root raw with your food, steep several slices in a pot of tea, or get it in capsule form. Add ginger to your diet gradually. If you're not used to it, ginger can cause a burning sensation in your mouth or stomach.

Spinach. If you suffer from migraines, chances are you don't have enough magnesium in your system. This might explain why nearly 80 percent of 3,000 migraine sufferers reported migraine relief after taking 200 milligrams (mg) of magnesium a day. If you choose to boost your magnesium intake, don't take more than 500 mg a day in supplement form. You can get plenty of magnesium in foods like spinach, potatoes, fish and shellfish, beans, and cereal.

Mushrooms. These fleshy buttons have relatively high levels of riboflavin, or vitamin B2. In one three-month study, people who took 400 mg of vitamin B2 a day had 37 percent fewer migraines than those given a placebo. While you can purchase riboflavin supplements in health food stores, you can also get modest amounts of vitamin B2 from spinach, cereals, liver, yogurt, milk, and cottage cheese.

Fortified milk. Milk is rich in both calcium and vitamin D – a combination that may keep migraines few and far between. Two women with severe migraines took megadoses of vitamin D and calcium and noticed their headaches came dramatically less often. Doctors think that low levels of these nutrients can bring on migraines. High doses of vitamin D can be dangerous, but you can get moderate amounts from milk, shrimp, and salmon. Good sources of calcium include milk products, greens, broccoli, and oysters.

Though not guaranteed to ward off all headaches, a meal rich in these nutrients can nip some migraines in the bud. And if you have migraines, even a little relief counts.

Pull migraine triggers from your diet

Want to diffuse a migraine before it starts? If you know what sets you off, you can. Here are some common foods that can cause trouble.

Watch out for soy. A man who ate lots of soy for his prostate mysteriously developed migraines. Once he cut back on the soy, they went away. Experts think that because soy has natural compounds that act like estrogen, it may trigger a migraine. If you are prone to headaches, keep your soy portions small.

Cut the fat. A low-fat diet will not only improve your figure – it can banish headaches as well. High levels of fat in your blood may encourage the blood vessels in your head to expand and bring on a migraine. In a recent California study, 42 women and 12 men managed to lower their dietary fat intake to 20 grams a day. They had fewer migraines and lighter symptoms.

If this low-fat diet leaves you hungry, fill up on vegetables, fruit, and beans. This winning combination of nutrients may also help you sidestep a migraine.

Say no to chocolate. This sweet treat, along with alcohol, aged cheese, caffeine, and processed meats, may trigger a migraine. Food additives and preservatives are other possible culprits.

Different foods affect different people. If you don't already know what triggers your migraines, keep a food diary to track it down. It might be as elusive as the scent of oranges on someone's skin or the artificial sweetener in your medicine.

Healthy habits

Try these tips to prevent and relieve tension headaches.

- Eat regular meals. Skipping meals or going a long time between meals can trigger a headache.
- Sit up straight. Poor posture can lead to tight neck and shoulder muscles, which contribute to headaches.
- Take a quick nap.
- Put two tennis balls in a sock. Lie on your back and wedge the balls behing your neck, one on each side. The gentle pressure can relieve your tension.
- Heat up salt in a dry pan until it's warm but not hot. Wrap the salt in a thin towel. Rub the warm pack on the back of your head to draw out the pain.
- Drink plenty of water. Dehydration causes headaches.
- Add a teaspoon of powdered mustard or ginger to a tub of hot water. Soak your feet for head-to-toe relief.

- Relax in a steamy bath with an ice pack on your head.
- Speak with a counselor, friend, or pastor. Talking about your problems can ease tension.

CHAPTER 16

Heartburn & indigestion

What is heartburn and indigestion? Indigestion simply means poor digestion. Acid indigestion, or heartburn, occurs when your stomach contents back up into your esophagus, the tube that carries food down your throat.

Who gets it? As many as 60 million Americans suffer from it monthly, and 25 million have it daily.

What are the symptoms?

- burning in your chest or throat, or chest pain, especially after eating or lying down
- sour taste in your mouth, bad breath, lump in your throat, difficulty swallowing, chronic hoarseness, sore throat, wheezing, or night cough
- belching, nausea, or vomiting

Sensible solutions to heartburn

You may have seen those drug commercials that say heartburn can have serious long-term complications. That's not just a sales ploy. Acid indigestion over time can cause bleeding and ulcers in your esophagus, a precancerous condition called Barrett's esophagus, and even asthma. But you don't need medicines to prevent these complications. A natural mix of healthy foods and eating habits will set you on your way to heartburn-free living.

If you have frequent heartburn — a symptom of gastroesophageal reflux disease (GERD) — it's because the ring of muscles between your esophagus and stomach doesn't work properly. "There's supposed to be a one-way valve," explains Dr. Timothy C. Wang, chief of the Division of Gastroenterology at the

University of Massachusetts Medical School. "Food is supposed to go down, but nothing really much is supposed to come up. But in people who have problems with GERD, that one-way valve is a little loose."

Food and stomach acids then back up into your throat, causing the all-too familiar symptoms of heartburn. In some cases, basic changes in your diet may be all you need to overcome them.

Find the right fat ratio. First, heartburn experts recommend limiting fat to less than 30 percent of your diet. But more importantly, know which fats to keep and which to toss. "The main thing is the fat content," Wang advises. "High fat food. Fried foods with a lot of butter and oil. These seem to precipitate heartburn."

That means, say bye-bye to cream and meat sauces and soups, butter, margarine, meats, cheese, pizza, fried foods, mayo, and other sources of unhealthy saturated fats. If you can't bear to give up these foods, replace them with low-fat versions.

Drop the pounds. One recent study from Europe emphasized what most experts have suggested all along – being overweight is an acid indigestion instigator. Extra weight seems to put stress on that one-way valve and cause it to malfunction.

Losing weight is easier said than done, you say? But you're halfway there when you avoid saturated fats and limit total fat intake to less than 30 percent. A recent Harvard study found those steps may help people lose weight better than a strict low-fat diet.

The Harvard diet also calls for you to beef up your intake of healthier unsaturated fats. These include the omega-3 fatty acids in fish, flaxseed, and walnuts, and the monounsaturated fats in nuts, peanut butter, and olives.

Cut down on calories. Eating fewer calories is definitely a tried-and-true weight-loss strategy. On its own, it could be a way to control your heartburn, according to groundbreaking research from Europe.

In this study, researchers tested a low-fat, high-calorie meal versus a low-calorie meal. Those eating fewer calories suffered fewer episodes of reflux over the next four hours. The low-calorie food appeared to decrease stomach acid and leave the stomach more quickly. In the process, the one-way valve closed up faster. Although a small study, the results suggest eating a low-calorie meal maybe a strategy worth trying.

Fill your plate with fiber. "One of the things that worsens heartburn is any degree of constipation," Wang says. "Treating constipation sometimes – not always – can alleviate or reduce heartburn."

Munching on fiber-filled foods is proven to help you get regular. And though this may not do the trick for your heartburn, fruits, vegetables, and whole grains at least can fill you up without weighing you down – and weighing down your scale. That's because high-fiber foods have a lot of volume without a lot of calories.

Chase it with water. Make sure to get your daily six to eight glasses of water while you're at it. Like a sponge, fiber will absorb the water and swell, making you feel even fuller. The water will also help your body cope with the side effects of fiber, like constipation and gas. On top of that, water itself is a good remedy for heartburn. It clears your throat and dilutes the acid in your stomach.

With these changes, you'll still have variety in your diet and get the same pleasure from eating. Only you may have less heartburn and a smaller waistline, too. Just be aware that if the changes don't help, you may have something more serious, like a damaged esophagus or internal bleeding. According to Dr.

Loren Laine, professor of medicine at the University of Southern California, symptoms such as difficulty swallowing, pain with swallowing, bleeding (i.e., vomiting blood, black stools, or iron-deficiency anemia), or weight loss, are cause for concern. "Alarm symptoms," he warns, "should prompt early medical evaluation rather than just treating the symptoms of GERD."

Otherwise, you could end up as a statistic in one of those heartburn commercials.

Stamp out heartburn with spicy foods

Look in your kitchen, not your medicine cabinet, to heal your heartburn and indigestion. Surprisingly, some spicy foods may help put out the fire in your belly. But you'll also find soothing relief in other foods and drinks as well.

Take a chance on chili peppers. A hot jalapeno may be the last thing you think of grabbing when your stomach is on the fritz, but it actually may be one of the best. The active ingredient in chili peppers, capsaicin, works wonders on a stomach. It increases blood flow, gets digestive juices running, moves the muscles of your digestive system, and dispels gas.

Still, a fiery bowl of chili is not to be taken lightly. Too much capsaicin can give you an even bigger bellyache. So talk with your doctor before making hot peppers a regular part of your diet. If she gives you the green light, try them in small doses first to see how your stomach reacts.

Add a dash of cinnamon. The ancient Greeks and Romans gave us democracy and the Olympics. So why not follow their lead when it comes to indigestion and add cinnamon to your food? Heartburn sufferers in ancient times relied on the spice to help their digestion. Today's experts aren't exactly sure how it works, but they suspect it may have something to do with how cinnamon heats up your stomach.

Sprinkle on turmeric. One of the world's leading voices in herbal medicine, the German Commission E, touts this exotic spice as a cure for indigestion. Turmeric seems to prompt your liver to pump out more bile, an essential digestive fluid. If you don't have enough bile, you'll feel dyspeptic – bloated and sick to your stomach – after a normal-sized meal.

You can get more turmeric in your diet by eating curry dishes because it's a key ingredient. But you can also find the pure spice in your grocery store. Try sprinkling a half tablespoon on your food every day to help avoid that bloated, uncomfortable feeling. But talk to your doctor first before you begin treating yourself. Turmeric is strong enough stuff that you should avoid it if you have certain conditions, like a gallstone.

Savor the zing of ginger. This herb doesn't monkey around with indigestion either. It's on the German Commission E's list of powerful natural aids for heartburn and bloating. The Commission recommends eating a 1-inch chunk of ginger every day. Add it to a stir fry or make ginger tea. To brew this tasty beverage, grate the ginger and steep it in hot water for 10 minutes. You can also buy ginger supplements. The recommended dosage is 500 to 1,000 milligrams a day.

Enjoy the power of yogurt. You normally don't want to invite bacteria into your belly. But in the case of this dairy food, you do. Yogurt helps build up your stomach's good bacteria, and these bacateria are key for proper digestion. Yogurt even can work for lactose intolerant people, since its bacteria digest the milk sugar for you. For best results, buy plain yogurt that contains active cultures. Then stir in your own fresh fruit.

Rely on bananas for relief. Don't get choked up over the dry cough you have from your chronic heartburn. Bananas are a great remedy for this common side effect of acid indigestion. Eat them whole, or buy banana powder at your local health food store.

Experiment with artichokes. Like turmeric, artichoke leaves encourage your liver to produce more bile, which may keep you from feeling bloated and full.

Avoid heartburn triggers like caffeinated drinks, tomato-based foods, citrus fruit, onions, peppers, chocolate, and mints. Limit sodas and sweet treats, too. All their sugar can cause a bellyache.

If artichokes don't make the grade in your book, try one of the other "bitters," such as watercress, dandelion leaves, endive, or grated orange peels. Just like their artichoke cousin, these plants can get your digestive juices flowing.

Soothe your stomach with sparkling water. According to a new study from Europe, seltzer also helps wash away dyspepsia. For two weeks, participants drank about 1.5 quarts of either tap water or carbonated water each day. Those who drank the sparkling water found their indigestion had improved, and they suffered less constipation. Alhough the study was small, it can't hurt to switch to carbonated water for your six glasses a day and see if it helps.

Relax with chamomile tea. This soothing flower has been known since ancient time as a cure for an upset stomach and indigestion. Look for dried chamomile at your local health food store. Steep a heaping teaspoon in hot water for 15 minutes. Then drink a cup between meals three or four times a day.

Take the fright out of severe chest pain

You suddenly feel excruciating chest pain, and thinking the worst, you race to the emergency room. But in the end, you find out it isn't a heart attack — just a bad case of heartburn.

This frightening and embarrassing situation happens to millions of people every year, making heartburn the leading cause of unexplained chest pain. But you can avoid becoming another statistic by managing your heartburn with your doctor's help.

"GERD (gastroesophageal reflux disease) is the most common abnormality associated with unexplained chest pain," says Dr. Philip O. Katz, chairman of the Department of Medicine at Philadelphia's Graduate Hospital. "The important thing is for sufferers to speak to their physicians at the onset of symptoms."

You should be checked for GERD if you have heartburn more than twice a week, frequent coughing, difficulty swallowing, or a bad aftertaste in your mouth. By discussing these symptoms with your doctor, you will be better prepared for severe episodes and less likely to make that scary trip to the ER.

Signs that your chest pain may actually be a heart attack include nausea, sweating, weakness, breathlessness, fainting, or shooting pain from your jaw to your arm. If you experience those symptoms, don't hesitate to get emergency treatment, says Dr. Robert W. Schafermeyer, president of the American College of Emergency Physicians.

"It is right for anyone with severe abdominal or chest pain to seek immediate emergency medical treatment," he says. "However," he adds, "there is much fear and anxiety related to severe chest pain that could be prevented if a person works with their doctor to prevent GERD emergencies."

Healthy habits

To avoid heartburn symptoms, you may have to change your usual habits. According to Dr. Timothy Wang, these are "standard lifestyle modifications" that all heartburn sufferers should follow.

- Don't eat before bedtime. Don't even lie down for four hours after eating.
- Eat small meals throughout the day rather than eating three big ones.

- Chew your food well. Take smaller bites.
- Don't work or drive while eating. Sit straight and dine.
- Allow an hour before and after eating before you drink any liquids.
- Drink plenty in between meals, especially when you are taking medications.
- Enjoy sugar-free candy after meals to get saliva going. Saliva neutralizes stomach acids.
- Lose weight if you're overweight.
- Quit smoking and limit alcohol.
- Wear loose clothing.
- Ask your doctor whether the medications you are taking could cause heartburn.
- Raise the head of your bed 6 inches.
- Sleep on your left side, which seems to be the best position for preventing heartburn.
- Avoid heavy lifting and straining.

For frequent heartburn, these tips aren't enough. "If heartburn's happening more than twice a week," Wang warns, "you should seek medical attention."

CHAPTER 17

Hiatal hernia

What is a hiatal hernia? It's when your stomach pokes through a tear in your diaphragm, the sheet of muscle between your stomach and chest. The diaphragm can act like a vice around the top part of your stomach, holding digestive juices there longer than usual and bringing on heartburn and pain.

Who gets it? Hiatal hernia is common in people age 50 and older, even in those who are otherwise healthy.

What are the symptoms? Sometimes there aren't any. Otherwise, they may include:

- heartburn or a sour taste in your mouth
- bloating, belching, or vomiting
- discomfort or pain in your throat or stomach

Secret for preventing hiatal hernia

The late Dr. Denis Burkitt had it right over 20 years ago. Burkitt, a surgeon who pioneered the study of fiber, claimed that a roughage-rich diet could prevent and treat hiatal hernias.

Though today's experts aren't 100 percent sure, they believe straining from coughing, vomiting, or overexerting yourself can cause a hiatal hernia. Burkitt saw constipation as another source of this straining.

He proved his point with statistics. One in five middle-age Americans in Burkitt's day had a hiatal hernia. On the other hand, Burkitt found only one in 250 African adults with the condition. The reason for this huge gap, he explained, was the difference in people's diets.

> **Here are two tricks to help you get more fiber from fruits and vegetables — choose raw or lightly cooked produce, and whenever you can, eat the skin.**

Simply put, the Africans ate more than their fair share of fiber, while the Americans didn't – and still don't.

The National Academies' Institute of Medicine recommends men age 50 and over get 30 grams of fiber a day. Women of the same age need 21 grams. According to recent reports, Americans eat as little as 5 grams. No wonder over 4 million people complain they're constipated on a regular basis, and many more have hiatal hernias.

There are two different kinds of fiber, and it's important to increase your intake of both. Yet, to reduce the pressures of constipation and prevent a hiatal hernia, zero in on the insoluble kind.

- **Insoluble.** This is the roughage your grandmother used to talk about. Think thick vegetable skins, husks, and kernels, which travel through your digestive system without being digested. In the process, this fiber speeds up the passage of your bowel movements by making them soft and easy to pass. Foods high in insoluble fiber include whole grains, wheat bran, fruits, vegetables, seeds, legumes, brown rice, and popcorn.

- **Soluble.** This kind of fiber dissolves into a gel-like substance in your digestive tract and soaks up extra cholesterol and keeps blood sugar levels under control. Sources of soluble fiber include fruits, vegetables, seeds, rye, oats, barley, rice bran, and legumes.

It's important to increase your fiber gradually over the course of several weeks. In addition, make sure to drink enough water and other fluids. These steps will help you avoid the side effects of a high-fiber diet, such as even more constipation, gas, and bloating.

Healthy habits

Hiatal hernias are so common in seniors they may seem like a fact of life. Still, you don't need to put up with their side effects. Make these simple lifestyle changes to calm the symptoms.

- Stop smoking.
- Lose weight if you're overweight.
- Schedule several small meals throughout the day instead of a few big ones.
- Don't eat two to three hours before bedtime.
- Limit caffeinated and alcoholic drinks, as well as mint, chocolate, citrus fruits, tomato products, and fried foods.
- Sit upright while eating and remain that way for one hour after a meal.
- Raise the head of your bed 6 inches.
- Wear loose clothing.

CHAPTER 18 *High blood pressure*

What is high blood pressure? Blood pressure is the force of your blood pushing against your arteries. You suffer from high blood pressure, or hypertension, when your heart must work harder than normal to pump blood through your circulatory system. This can damage both your heart and arteries and boost your risk of heart attack, stroke, kidney failure, eye damage, congestive heart failure, and atherosclerosis.

Who gets high blood pressure? People over 60 and blacks are at greater risk. Being overweight and inactive, smoking, drinking, stress, and a diet high in salt and fat can also contribute.

What are the symptoms? There are no outer symptoms. The main warning sign is a blood pressure reading higher than 140/90.

Eat your way to lower blood pressure

Food does more than fill you up and taste good. It can also have a major impact on your heart. If you're concerned about high blood pressure, the right menu can make a big difference.

Read on to get the latest word on what you should and shouldn't eat. The following foods will give you the maximum blood pressure benefits.

Fruits and vegetables. Think of fruits and vegetables as nature's magic pills, containing lots of vitamins and minerals that help your heart. A recent British study determined that boosting your fruit and vegetable intake to the recommended five servings a day can dramatically lower your blood pressure. The increased potassium from a produce-rich diet probably had the biggest effect on blood pressure. But people in the study also boosted levels of antioxidant vitamins like vitamin C and beta carotene.

When calculating your intake of fruits and vegetables, remember a serving equals one medium-size piece of fruit or half a cup of cooked veggies.

University of California-Berkeley professor Gladys Block and her colleagues recently conducted a study to determine how vitamin C affects blood pressure. Quite simply, low levels of vitamin C in your blood can mean high blood pressure. Oranges and broccoli, which were used in the study, are two great sources of vitamin C. Eat a wide variety of fruits and vegetables to make your menu more exciting – and healthy.

Whole grains. You don't have to battle high blood pressure – a muffin can drop it like a rock. Just make sure the muffin is made with healthy whole grains, like oats. Researchers at the University of Minnesota found that eating fiber-rich, whole-grain oat cereal can significantly lower blood pressure.

In fact, 73 percent of the people in the study were able to cut back on their blood pressure medication. The soluble fiber in oats did the trick. People in the study ate about three-fourths of a cup of Quaker Oatmeal and a cup and a third of Quaker Oat Squares each day.

Fish. Several studies note fish's ability to lower blood pressure. The secret? Omega-3 fatty acids. These fats help widen, rather than narrow, your blood vessels. They also keep your blood from clumping and sticking. That way, your heart doesn't have to work as hard.

You should try to eat several fatty fish meals every week. Salmon, mackerel, herring, and tuna are your best bets. You can also find omega-3 in walnuts, flaxseed, and collard and turnip greens.

Olive oil. Halt high blood pressure with this food, a flavorful oil that's perfect for cooking and salad dressings. People in a recent Italian study significantly lowered their blood pressure after eating a diet rich in extra-virgin olive oil for six months. Olive oil was so powerful they were able to cut their dosage of blood pressure lowering medication almost in half. Keep in mind the diet was also low in total and saturated fat.

Pumpkin seed oil. If you take medication for your high blood pressure, you might also want to take some pumpkin seed oil. A Saudi Arabian study of rats found that pumpkin seed oil may improve the effectiveness of calcium antagonists and ACE-inhibitors. Rich in the antioxidants vitamin E and selenium, pumpkin seed oil is available in capsule form, as well as a nutty-flavored oil you can use for salad dressings.

Just as some foods can help lower your blood pressure, others pose a danger. When planning your menu, remember to forget these blood pressure boosting items.

Salt. This is the big one. You're probably already aware of salt's negative effect on blood pressure. But now there's new proof. A recent Johns Hopkins study found that reducing sodium, a component of salt, helps older people lower their blood pressure and control high blood pressure. Those who cut back on salt also had fewer headaches and episodes of angina.

> **Gobble guava and lower your blood pressure, according to an Indian study. This tasty fruit, high in potassium and soluble fiber, can be found fresh, canned, and in pastes, juices, jams, and jellies.**

Saturated fat. Limit red meat, butter, and whole milk products. This helps not only your blood pressure, but your all-around heart health.

Alcohol. Drink only in moderation. Large amounts of alcohol can wreak havoc on your blood pressure. Men should have no more than two drinks a day. And for women, no more than one drink a day.

Licorice. This treat plays tricks on your blood pressure. Because of an ingredient called glycyrrhizic acid, licorice causes your body to retain sodium and fluids and lose potassium. Fortunately, only real licorice has this effect. Most of the licorice sold in the United States is made with artificial flavoring, usually anise.

Be on the lookout for real licorice in unexpected places, such as tobacco products and laxatives.

Caffeine. A University of Oklahoma study found that caffeine, when taken during stressful situations, can boost high blood pressure even higher.

In some cases, the blood pressure remained high 12 hours after a single dose of caffeine. Researchers from Greece and Australia determined that caffeine may also stiffen your arteries and further raise blood pressure in those with high blood pressure. If you don't have high blood pressure, a coffee break won't hurt. But if you do, consider taking a break from coffee.

Sugar. Sweets and sugar-containing drinks provide plenty of calories, but little nutritional value. Not to mention the extra calories they sneak into your diet. Remember, keeping your weight under control also helps keep your blood pressure under control.

Spice up your life without salt

Variety might be the spice of life – but when was the last time you sprinkled some variety on your food? Unfortunately for your blood pressure, salt seems to be the true spice of life.

Salt, also known as sodium chloride, is an important mineral that is 40 percent sodium and 60 percent chloride. The average American takes in between 4,000 and 6,000 milligrams (mg) of sodium a day, well above the recommended 2,400 mg. Fortunately, you can take simple steps to cut back on salt, lower your blood pressure, and still enjoy a delicious meal.

Skimp on processed food. Some people are more sensitive to salt than others. For these people, reducing salt intake drastically lowers blood pressure. Those who fall in this category, according to a recent analysis of the Dietary Approaches to Stop Hypertension (DASH)-Sodium Trial, include people with high blood pressure, blacks, women, and people older than 45.

But restricting salt helps everyone lower blood pressure. That's why it's a good idea to limit your sodium intake to 2,400 mg, or about one teaspoon of salt, a day.

Don't heap all the blame on your salt shaker. Processed foods, such as frozen dinners, restaurant meals, and canned foods, contribute the most salt in your diet. If you cut down on those foods and limit the salt you use while cooking and at the table, you'll be on your way to lower blood pressure.

> Japanese scientists have discovered the enzyme responsible for making you cry when you cut an onion. Now they're looking into ways to remove the enzyme, but not the flavor.

Won't your food taste bland without salt? Not if you make some smart – and delicious – substitutions. Here are some healthy alternatives to salt.

Grab some garlic. The ancient Chinese used this fragrant bulb to fight high blood pressure, and scientific studies have shown this spice lowers blood pressure and cholesterol.

While recent studies aren't as conclusive regarding its heart-protective powers, garlic still adds flavor without contributing to high blood pressure. DASH even recommends cooking with garlic and onions as flavorful alternatives to salt.

Squeeze a lemon. Garlic and onions are only the beginning. Lemon, lime, vinegar, and many herbs and spices give your food amazing flavor without the danger that comes with salt.

Check out these creative ways the American Heart Association suggests to spice up your meals.

- **Fish** – basil, curry powder, dill, garlic, lemon juice, dry mustard, nutmeg, paprika, parsley, sage, or turmeric.

- **Chicken** – curry powder, dill, ginger, dry mustard, nutmeg, or rosemary.

- **Lean meats** – allspice, bay leaves, caraway seeds, chives, curry powder, garlic, lemon juice, dry mustard, onion, paprika, parsley, sage, thyme, or turmeric.

- **Soups** – basil, bay leaves, caraway seeds, chives, dill, garlic, onions, paprika, parsley, or thyme.

- **Stews** – allspice, basil, bay leaves, caraway seeds, or sage.

- **Sauces** – basil, chives, cider vinegar, dry mustard, paprika, parsley, rosemary, thyme, or turmeric.

- **Vegetables** – chives, cider vinegar, garlic, lemon juice, onion, paprika, or parsley.

Experiment with new flavors. Your heart and your taste buds will thank you. After all, a little variety never hurt anyone.

Beware of pain relievers

Many health experts often recommend low-dose aspirin therapy for your heart. But research shows its effect on blood pressure remains unclear.

Maybe timing is everything. A small Spanish study found that people with mild high blood pressure who took their low-dose aspirin before bed lowered their blood pressure much more than those who took it when they awoke or eight hours after waking.

Unfortunately, not all pain relievers bring relief to your heart. A new study links high blood pressure to frequent use of common over-the-counter pain relievers. These include acetaminophen (Tylenol) and NSAIDs, like ibuprofen (Advil, Motrin) or naproxen (Aleve).

People who took acetaminophen 22 days a month or more doubled their chances of developing high blood pressure. Those who took NSAIDs that often were 86 percent more likely to have high blood pressure.

This is the first study to find such a link, and more research is needed. So you don't need to stop taking pain relievers – but if you take them often, have your blood pressure checked regularly.

Manage blood pressure with minerals

Three's a crowd – except when it comes to fighting high blood pressure. That's when you need the powerful triple threat of potassium, magnesium, and calcium.

You can drop your blood pressure like a rock with this trio of minerals found in these foods.

Go bananas for potassium. If you're battling high blood pressure, you probably know all about the perils of salt. But potassium plays just as big a role in controlling blood pressure.

Study after study shows that adding potassium to your diet helps lower blood pressure. This strategy has a greater benefit for people with elevated blood pressure, but even those with normal blood pressure may see an improvement. The combination of adding potassium and limiting salt has an even greater effect.

While its main asset is its ability to control blood pressure, that's not all potassium does. Potassium is a miracle mineral that not only helps lower blood pressure and cholesterol but has at least seven other heart-healthy benefits. They include:

- protecting your blood vessels from damage

- preventing dangerous irregular heartbeats

- reducing your risk of stroke

- dilating blood vessels

- suppressing renin, an enzyme produced by your kidneys that contributes to high blood pressure

- prompting your sympathetic nervous system to regulate blood pressure

- prodding your kidneys to get rid of more sodium and less calcium through your urine

> **A banana gives you 467 milligrams (mg) of potassium. But a half cup of dried apricots gives you about 900 mg.**

It's easy to boost your potassium intake. Good sources of potassium include peas, beans, apricots, peaches, bananas, prunes, oranges, spinach, stewed tomatoes, sweet potatoes, avocados, and figs.

Go nuts for magnesium. Consider magnesium one of potassium's henchmen in the fight against high blood pressure. This mineral relaxes blood vessels and balances the potassium and sodium in your blood cells.

A four-year study of more than 30,000 men found that getting more magnesium into your diet was significantly associated with a lower risk of high blood pressure. In fact, the Joint National Committee on Prevention, Detection, Evaluation, and Treatment of High Blood Pressure recommends maintaining an adequate magnesium intake as a way to prevent and manage high blood pressure.

Food sources of magnesium include whole-wheat breads and cereals, broccoli, chard, spinach, okra, oysters, scallops, sea bass, mackerel, beans, nuts, and seeds.

Say cheese for calcium. As you get older, your systolic blood pressure, the top number in a blood pressure reading, tends to go up. A recent University of South Carolina study found that boosting your calcium intake may help slow this increase.

Calcium helps control blood pressure by helping your body get rid of sodium through your urine. Previous studies have shown that people who don't get much calcium in their diet often have high blood pressure.

You can find calcium in cheese, milk, yogurt, broccoli, spinach, turnip greens, mackerel, perch, and salmon.

Make an effort to include plenty of potassium, magnesium, and calcium in your diet. When you see the effect on your blood pressure, you'll agree that three's company.

Healthy habits

Just because you've left the table doesn't mean you can call a cease-fire in the war against high blood pressure.

Try these natural ways to lower your blood pressure and reduce stress.

- Exercise regularly. Just walking an extra mile or two each day can help. Find ways to add steps to your day, such as taking the stairs instead of the elevator or parking at the rear of a parking lot.

- Maintain a normal body weight. Aim to lose weight if you're overweight.

- Limit alcohol. Binge drinking is more harmful than regular, moderate drinking.

- Quit smoking.
- Listen to music to relax.
- Get a pet. A loving cat or dog can do wonders for your blood pressure.
- Spend time with your spouse or a close friend. You'll feel safe, comfortable, and less stressed.
- Control your anger. For your heart's sake, try to look at the positive side of every situation.

CHAPTER 19 *High cholesterol*

What is high cholesterol? Your body needs cholesterol to build cell walls and make hormones. But too much of this soft, waxy substance can be deadly. It builds up on your artery walls, causing blockages that lead to heart attack or stroke. Low-density lipoprotein (LDL) is called bad cholesterol because it carries cholesterol to your arteries. High-density lipoprotein (HDL) is the good guy that transports cholesterol to your liver, where it is eliminated.

Who gets it? Overweight, inactive people, smokers, and those who eat lots of saturated fat get high cholesterol. Older people and diabetics are at greater risk, and family history also plays a role.

What are the symptoms? No outer symptoms. Total cholesterol over 200 mg/dl; LDL levels over 130 mg/dl; HDL under 40 mg/dl.

Fight back with flaxseed and nuts

Manufacturers constantly sneak extra fat, sugar, and sodium into your food. But you can be just as sneaky in order to protect your heart. Just make room in your diet for flaxseed and nuts, two tiny but powerful weapons against high cholesterol.

Give flaxseed a whirl. The seeds from the flax plant amazingly lower your cholesterol levels and your blood pressure at the same time. Loaded with soluble fiber that lowers cholesterol, flaxseed is also the best plant source of omega-3 fatty acids.

These fats, found mainly in fish, keep your blood from sticking, regulate your heartbeat, and lower your blood pressure. They've also been shown to lower cholesterol.

Whether because of the soluble fiber, omega-3 fatty acids, or some other ingredient, flaxseed works. Studies have shown flaxseed can lower cholesterol by as much as 14.7 percent. Just remember, to get the benefits, you must grind up the seeds first.

About 95 percent of U.S. flax is grown in North Dakota. Right now, researchers at North Dakota State University are busy developing flax pasta and flax ice cream.

It's easy to sneak flaxseed into your diet. Here's an instant way to keep your arteries free of clogging plaque. Just whip flaxseed up in your smoothies. You can also mix ground flaxseed into oatmeal, rice pilaf, applesauce, or yogurt. Or add it to salads, soups, cereals, and baked goods.

For example, bake some flaxseed bread. This amazing bread works exactly like cholesterol-lowering drugs, but without the side effects. One study found that people who ate six slices of flaxseed bread a day significantly lowered their cholesterol.

More good news. This tasty little seed fights cholesterol and cancer. Researchers are recognizing it to be a tiny double powerhouse in disease prevention. When you eat flaxseed, you not only protect your heart, you also guard against breast, prostate, and colon cancers. Introduce flaxseed to your diet gradually. If you add too much too quickly, you might experience digestive problems, like gas.

Go nuts. Nuts are another good way to get good fats into your diet. In fact, eating more nuts can save your life. Studies have shown that eating nuts at least five times a week can slash your risk of heart attack in half.

Here are some tasty nuts worth nibbling.

- Walnuts, another good source of omega-3 fatty acids, have been proven to lower cholesterol. Like many nuts, walnuts are also high in antioxidant vitamin E.

- Pecans, rich in heart-healthy monounsaturated fat, helped reduce total cholesterol by 6.7 percent and LDL cholesterol by 10.4 percent in a recent study.

- Almonds, featuring monounsaturated fat, protein, and fiber, helped lower cholesterol in two recent studies.

Like flaxseed, nuts are easy to add to your diet. Sprinkle them in salads or cereals, add them to baked goods, or just grab a handful for a healthy snack. But don't forget – when you eat nuts, be sure to cut calories elsewhere.

Foil cholesterol with these delicious foods

Like a comic book villain, cholesterol has hatched a sinister plot to take over the world – or at least your arteries. Soluble fiber to the rescue. This mighty superhero, found in fruits, vegetables, and cereals, can gum up the works and foil cholesterol's evil schemes. Here's how it works.

Pick an apple. Unlike money, apples grow on trees. That's great news for your heart. This common, inexpensive, high-pectin fruit can lower your cholesterol by up to 30 percent if you eat it every day.

> **You can lower your cholesterol just by using non-fat milk instead of whole milk, which has seven times more cholesterol and 19 times more saturated fat.**

Pectin, a gummy form of soluble fiber, has been shown to lower cholesterol. That's because it binds with harmful LDL cholesterol and carries it out of your body. And that's not all it does. It also relieves constipation and diarrhea.

Pectin isn't all that apples have going for them. Apples also contain vitamin C, the minerals magnesium and potassium to help regulate blood pressure, and flavonoids like quercetin that act as antioxidants. It all adds up to a very powerful piece of fruit.

An apple a day might keep the doctor away. But, according to a French study, eating two apples a day can lower your cholesterol by as much as 30 percent.

Sow some oats. Use some good, old-fashioned horse sense, and eat more oats. Oats feature beta-glucan, another form of soluble fiber. Like pectin, beta-glucan is sticky. This stickiness helps slow down the movement of food through your stomach and small intestine, giving HDL particles more time to pick up cholesterol. That means you reduce the chances that cholesterol will be carried by LDL particles to your artery walls.

> **Psyllium is another FDA-recommended soluble fiber. It's sold as a laxative, like Metamucil, or as a powder and can also be found in some cereals.**

Two recent studies determined that adding two servings of oats, either in the form of oatmeal or oat bran cereal, can reduce your cholesterol.

In fact, the FDA recommends getting four servings of foods containing beta-glucan each day to reduce the risk of cardiovascular disease. One serving of beta-glucan equals .75 grams, so four servings would total 3 grams. Foods meeting that requirement can display this heart-healthy claim.

Many health experts recommend getting between 20 and 35 grams of fiber a day, and it doesn't all have to come from oats. You can get fiber from fruits and vegetables, too. But consider increasing your cereal fiber. This powerful healing food can save your life.

In a Harvard study of fiber intake, men who ate the most cereal fiber drastically lowered their risk of heart disease. The more they ate, the more their cholesterol came down. For every 10-gram increase in cereal fiber, they slashed their risk of heart disease by nearly 30 percent. Start the day with a big bowl of high-fiber cereal, and you're on your way to a healthier heart.

Another great thing about fiber – and its trusty sidekick anti-oxidants – is you can find it in so many foods. That gives your menu both variety and punch.

So, gang up on cholesterol. Here are more delicious ways to bring it down and keep it down, from carrots to chocolate.

- **Prunes.** Lower your dangerous LDL cholesterol in just four weeks. This small, sweet fruit can help. In one study, men who ate 12 prunes a day, an amount that provides 6 grams of fiber, significantly lowered their LDL cholesterol.

- **Beans and legumes.** These staples are great – and cheap – sources of fiber.

- **Barley.** Like oats, barley contains cholesterol-lowering beta-glucan.

- **Pomegranate juice.** Loaded with antioxidants, this tangy beverage can prevent LDL oxidation, a necessary step in the development of atherosclerosis.

- **Cranberries.** These tart, high-fiber treats contain the most antioxidants of any fruit, according to a study by University of Scranton professor Joe Vinson. "Cranberries are one of the healthiest fruits. I think people should eat more of them," Vinson says. Drinking cranberry juice also helps prevent LDL oxidation.

> Honey is a smart substitute for sugar. Darker honey, like buckwheat honey, has greater anti-oxidant powers. A recent preliminary study found it can prevent LDL from being oxidized.

- **Carrots.** Crunch into a carrot, and reap the benefits of fiber and beta carotene, which your body turns into vitamin A. Studies have shown that beta carotene from foods, but not from supplements, can help your heart.

- **Chocolate.** Even chocolate in small amounts might help because it's chock-full of antioxidants. For more information on chocolate, please see *Shatter common cholesterol myths* on page 165.

With all these superheroes on your side, cholesterol doesn't stand a chance.

Exceptional way to eliminate bad cholesterol

It's an effective, easy, and exciting way to lower your cholesterol. It's also excellent, effortless, and economical. Give up? It's vitamin E, the powerful antioxidant vitamin that helps eliminate high cholesterol. Here's how it works and how you can get more of this important vitamin into your diet.

Some people are gentle until they have too much to drink. Then they get mean. That's kind of how LDL cholesterol is. Unless it becomes oxidized, it's pretty harmless. But once it's oxidized, it can collect on your artery walls, form plaques, and contribute to atherosclerosis. Vitamin E does its best to make sure LDL doesn't become oxidized.

Two recent studies determined vitamin E supplements can stop oxidation. But others have found a benefit only in getting vitamin E from whole foods. That's probably your best bet, because you can benefit from the food's other nutrients, too.

Arm yourself with wheat germ. This top-notch heart healer is packed with protein, fiber, polyunsaturated fatty acids, plant sterols, and plenty of vitamin E. You can dissolve cholesterol and open up arteries with just a quarter of a cup of wheat germ daily.

A French study found that eating 30 grams, or about a quarter of a cup, of raw wheat germ a day for 14 weeks lowered total cholesterol by 7.2 percent and LDL cholesterol by 15.4 percent. Vitamin E's antioxidant powers could be the reason for wheat germ's success. Other good food sources of vitamin E include nuts and seeds, vegetable oils, dark leafy greens, and whole grains.

Get friendly with olive oil. This flavorful oil, rich in vitamin E, monounsaturated fat, and other beneficial compounds, can be a tasty weapon against high cholesterol.

A recent Spanish study found that virgin olive oil increased LDL's resistance to oxidation, while a new Greek study determined that even the minor components of olive oil had major powers to stop LDL oxidation. Just 20 grams, or about a tablespoon and a half a day, of olive oil could help reduce your risk of heart disease.

How to boost your 'good' cholesterol

In life, you must take the good with the bad. Same with cholesterol. Don't just worry about lowering your LDL, or bad cholesterol. You can also take steps to boost your good HDL cholesterol levels. Remember, HDL protects your heart. It whisks cholesterol away from your arteries to your liver, where it's eliminated.

Try these 15 ways to raise your good cholesterol naturally and protect your heart and arteries.

- Snack on walnuts.

- Cook with olive oil and use it in salad dressings. It's a good source of heart-healthy monounsaturated fat.

- Bulk up on fiber. Cereals, legumes, fruits and vegetables, and whole-grain breads are good sources. Choose rye over wheat for best results.

- Boost your chromium intake. Sources include apples with skins, Brewer's yeast, fish and other seafood, mushrooms, liver, prunes, nuts, and asparagus.

- Sip alcohol in moderation – if you drink. Say when after one or two drinks.

- Eat more fish. Omega-3 fatty acids have been shown to raise HDL cholesterol.

- Add fresh garlic to your food.

- Drink orange juice. Three glasses a day can raise HDL by 21 percent, according to a Canadian study.

- Add calcium. Calcium citrate supplements raised HDL by 7 percent in older New Zealand women. Yogurt and low-fat dairy products are good food sources of calcium.

- Nibble on dark chocolate. According to a Penn State study, it not only slows LDL oxidation by 8 percent, it lifts HDL levels by 4 percent.

- Munch on a guava. An Indian study found adding guava to your diet can increase HDL levels by 8 percent.

- Exercise regularly.

- Lose weight if you are overweight.

- Give blood. Donating blood boosts your concentration of HDL, according to a South African study.

- Stop smoking.

If natural approaches don't work, your doctor can suggest some drug therapies to boost HDL. These include statins, niacin therapy, fibrates, and bile acid binding resins.

In the future, there might even be a cholesterol vaccine. It's still in the works, but keep your eyes open.

Maximize the power of statins

Your doctor may have prescribed a statin to help lower your cholesterol. Statins, like Zocor or Lipitor, do wonders for your cholesterol, but you can help them work even better. Here are effective strategies to help you maximize the power of statins.

Try the Mediterranean approach. A Finnish study found that eating a healthy diet and taking simvastatin (the generic name of Zocor) works better than either approach by itself.

People in the study ate a modified Mediterranean diet rich in omega-3 fatty acids. It featured fish, lean meats, low-fat dairy products, fruits, vegetables, cereals, and berries.

While simvastatin by itself lowered LDL cholesterol by 30 percent and the diet alone lowered LDL by 11 percent, the combination added up to a whopping 41 percent decrease.

The diet even counteracted some of simvastatin's side effects, including elevated insulin levels and depleted antioxidants.

Eat more often. This might sound like bizarre advice, but it's certainly worth a try. In a British study, people who ate six or more times a day had cholesterol levels about 5 percent lower than those who ate only once or twice.

This doesn't mean you should eat like a pig. Stick to a balanced diet, and split up your usual meals into smaller, more frequent ones. Choose healthy snacks, like fruits and nuts.

Foil fats with fish oil. An Australian study found another winning combination – fish oil capsules and atorvastatin (Lipitor). These things work in different ways to achieve a better balance of fats in your blood. While statins block the formation of cholesterol, fish oil stops the creation of triglycerides. Obese people with insulin resistance, which puts them at risk of developing diabetes, benefited from this dual treatment.

Follow new guidelines. The National Cholesterol Education Program recently announced new guidelines designed to help lower cholesterol levels.

Here are a few things, in addition to weight loss and increased physical activity, to keep in mind.

- Limit saturated fat to less than 7 percent of your total calories. Fat can account for up to one-third of your calories, as long as it's unsaturated.

- Keep cholesterol below 200 milligrams a day.

- Increase soluble fiber, the kind found in cereals and grains, to 10 to 25 grams a day.

- Add 2 grams of plant stanols or sterols a day. These natural, over-the-counter products, like Benecol or Take Control, can lower your cholesterol by 12 percent. Use them as a spread, like margarine.

Healthy habits

To lower your cholesterol, you'll need more than a healthy diet. Make the following steps part of your overall approach to a healthier heart.

- **Exercise.** Just 30 minutes a day of moderate exercise, such as brisk walking, slow jogging, or riding an exercise bike, can help lower LDL cholesterol.

- **Lose weight if you're overweight.** Maintain a healthy weight once you achieve it.

- **Stop smoking.**

- **Check your family history.** Knowing you might be at risk can give you an edge in prevention.

- **Get your cholesterol levels checked by a doctor.** You may need drug therapy.

Shatter common cholesterol myths

Surprise! When it comes to battling high cholesterol, some "evil" foods might not be villains after all. Check out these new spins on old enemies.

Crack the egg mystery. Perhaps you've been avoiding eggs because you're worried about your cholesterol. You must be "yolking." The American Heart Association says you can enjoy several eggs a week regardless of your cholesterol level. How many eggs does that add up to?

Studies show that eating up to one egg a day does not put you at greater risk for a heart attack or stroke, although an increase in heart disease risk was seen in diabetics.

Eggs do have lots of cholesterol, but they also provide healthy things – folate and other B vitamins; vitamins A, D, and E; protein; and monounsaturated fats. These helpful substances might counteract the damage done by the cholesterol.

A new Kansas State study sheds more light on the egg puzzle. Professor Sung I. Koo and colleagues found that a compound in eggs called lecithin reduces the amount of cholesterol your body absorbs.

"This may be a reason why so many studies found no association between egg intake and blood cholesterol," Koo says. "Less absorption means less cholesterol introduced into the blood.

We were able to determine experimentally that a substantial amount of egg cholesterol is not going into the bloodstream."

Part of the danger of eggs is that they go so well with bacon. People who eat a lot of eggs also tend to eat an unhealthy diet including bacon, red meat, whole milk, and few fruits and vegetables. A bad idea if you're watching your cholesterol.

Just in case its message about eggs got scrambled somewhere along the way, the American Heart Association recently clarified that an egg a day is OK – as long as you keep your total cholesterol to 300 mg or less.

Since an egg averages 213 mg of cholesterol, you'll have to limit your dietary cholesterol from other sources.

Scream for ice cream. Ice cream occupies a spot on every dieter's no-no list. But this delicious frozen treat has a secret weapon – guar gum.

Avoid guar gum diet pills. They can swell in your intestines, esophagus, or throat resulting in blockages or even death. Stick to guar gum in small, safe amounts in foods.

Guar gum, a form of soluble fiber, has been shown to lower cholesterol in numerous studies. In fact, adding gums to your diet can reduce LDL cholesterol by as much as 26 percent.

Manufacturers add guar gum to several foods to improve texture or bind various ingredients together. Some examples include soft drinks, baked goods, and salad dressings. You can also find this thickening agent in health food stores.

In ice cream, guar gum acts as a stabilizer to keep the ice cream smooth. Without it, ice cream would become coarse and icy very quickly.

Of course, you shouldn't go overboard on ice cream or mistake it for health food. It's still high in calories – and it's best to enjoy it sparingly. But next time you have a spoonful, remember guar gum, the secret ice cream ingredient that reduces LDL cholesterol by 26 percent.

Get sweet on chocolate. One of everyone's most craved treats has something to offer besides temptation and guilt. Along with great taste, chocolate also comes crammed with antioxidants called polyphenols.

Chocolate's polyphenols, similar to those found in vegetables and tea, can help your heart by preventing oxidation of LDL cholesterol. LDL cholesterol can harm your arteries when it becomes oxidized.

Here's another bonus that comes with eating chocolate. Cocoa and chocolate contain fats from cocoa butter. These fats are mostly stearic triglycerides, which are harder to absorb than other fats. That means they pass right through your body and have almost no effect on your cholesterol. And that's a pretty sweet deal.

This doesn't give you the green light to go hog wild eating chocolate. But a little chocolate, or some ice cream or an egg, now and then won't drive up your cholesterol.

CHAPTER 20

Insomnia

What is insomnia? Insomnia is the inability to fall asleep and stay asleep. It can lead to physical, mental, emotional, and safety problems.

Who gets it? People who are stressed or worried and those with sleep apnea or restless legs syndrome are prime candidates. Certain medications, too much light or noise in the bedroom, and too much caffeine can also keep you awake. Insomnia is especially common after age 65.

What are the symptoms?

- daytime drowsiness
- fatigue
- irritability
- difficulty coping

Fight fatigue with foods

Are you tired and drowsy all day from tossing and turning all night? The solution could be as simple as including the right nutrients in your diet.

You'll experience no more fatigue during the day, thanks to these four foods.

Wake up with cereal. Perhaps you start or end your day with a bowl of cereal because you know your body needs fiber. But did you know your brain needs it, too? According to a study at Cardiff University in Wales, people who regularly eat a high-fiber diet find it easier to fall asleep, enjoy a more positive mood, are less likely to be depressed, and are mentally sharper than those who eat a low-fiber diet.

Not all processed cereal is high in fiber, however. Check box labels for one with at least 5 grams per serving. Whole grains, like brown rice and bulgur, and fresh fruits and vegetables are other good high-fiber foods.

Step lively with beans. Magnesium, which helps your body produce sleep-regulating melatonin, is one good reason to eat beans. Tired all the time? Put the spring back in your step with this nutrient. A low level of magnesium – also found in nuts, green leafy vegetables, and whole grains – can result in both insomnia and fatigue.

Beans are high in brain-boosting fiber, too. Eat them plain or add them to soups and stews.

Sleep swimmingly with fish. Salmon and tuna are good sources of vitamin B3 and B6, both of which help your body make melatonin. Sunflower seeds and wheat bran also give you both of these vitamins. For additional vitamin B3, eat chicken, turkey, peanuts, and apricots. Get more B6 from avocados, bananas, carrots, rice, and shrimp.

Bounce back with chicken broth. Don't wait until you have a cold to enjoy soothing chicken soup. Have some, as well, when your brain is tired – like after doing your taxes or struggling to compare insurance policies.

Japanese researchers found a simple chicken extract can help you recover your energy more quickly after mental stress. A tasty bowl of soup should do the job even better.

Eat your way to sweet dreams

Life is like a bowl cherries when you feel rested. And cherries are just the sweet bedtime snack to open the door to restful sleep. That's because they contain lots of melatonin, a natural hormone that helps regulate your internal clock. It brings on the desire to sleep in darkness and triggers alertness in daylight.

As you get older, your body produces less melatonin. Nature, however, provides it through certain foods, and cherries seem to have the most. Eat a handful each night an hour or so before bedtime, and be prepared for pleasant dreams.

Forget counting sheep. A study at Oxford University found that imagining a waterfall or other relaxing scenes did a better job of bringing on sleep.

Experiment with other foods that contain melatonin – such as oats, sweet corn, rice, ginger, tomatoes, bananas, and barley – to find which ones work best for you. A banana smoothie or a bowl of tomato soup might be perfect for those nights when you aren't in the mood for cherries.

And there's more good news. Melatonin doesn't just help regulate your sleep. It's also an antioxidant that helps you fight heart disease, cancer, and a host of other ailments.

Top 10 healing herbs for insomnia

An old-time remedy for sleeplessness was to wash your head in a boiled dill seed solution before going to bed and to sniff this concoction from time to time during the night.

If that were the only way to get a good night's rest, it might be worth it. After all, getting too little sleep not only puts you in danger of having accidents, it also increases your risk of health problems like diabetes and high blood pressure.

Fortunately, using herbs can be easy and pleasant. It's one secret your pharmacist can't afford to tell you. The following herbs help you sleep – without the side effects of prescription sleep aids.

Valerian. This is one of the most popular, effective, and versatile herbs for conquering insomnia. Drink it in a tea, swallow it in a capsule, or add five to 10 drops of the aromatic oil to a relaxing bath.

Chamomile. Make a soothing cup of tea at bedtime to ease the stresses of the day. If you are allergic to pollen, however, choose a remedy other than this ragweed cousin.

Lavender. To soak away your cares before bedtime, add a few drops of lavender oil to a warm foot bath. Or light a lavender-scented candle and enjoy the calming aroma.

Hops. Stuff some of these dried fruits into a small sachet bag or pillow and place it inside your pillow case. Breathing the vapors from the alcohol in hops is probably what brings on the restful slumber.

Lemon balm. Sip a sleepy-time tea, or make a sachet pillow and inhale the soothing citrus scent.

Marjoram. For tranquil rest, add a bit of the aromatic oil to your evening bath.

Orange blossom. These flowers aren't just for brides. Place a bouquet beside your bed and let the fragrance take you gently into peaceful slumber.

Juniper. Sprinkle a few drops of the essential oil from this berry on a handkerchief and place it on your bedside table. As the aroma fills the air, you'll ease off to pleasant dreams.

Catnip. Cats seem to like the smell of this herb. People, however, tend to prefer the pleasant taste – and restful effects – of a cup of catnip tea before bedtime.

Passionflower. This flowering plant is particularly popular in England in preparations for calming the nerves. Brew a flavorful tea from the leaves and stems.

Not all herbs praised as sleep aids actually work, however. Some hyped-up herbs are even unsafe. Kava kava, for example, may do the job, but recent research shows a risk of liver damage with prolonged use. Skullcap, according to well-respected herbal expert Dr. Varro Tyler, is ineffective and may not be safe. And claims for linden flower are confusing. Some say it's a sedative, while others promote it as the opposite, a stimulant.

Many normally safe herbs can also be dangerous if you get too much. Because interactions sometimes cause problems, discuss their use with your doctor if you take prescription drugs, especially antidepressants.

Healthy habits

Conquer insomnia with these natural tips, and you'll wake up refreshed in the morning.

- Make friends. Lonely people don't sleep as well as those who are involved with others.
- Put pets in their own bed. They can disrupt your sleep if they share yours, leaving you dog-tired the next day.
- Go to bed and get up at the same time every day. Don't take naps.
- Keep your bedroom dark, quiet, and cool.
- Avoid caffeine in the afternoon or evening.
- Don't eat big meals before bedtime, but don't go to bed hungry, either.
- Get regular exercise, but not late in the day.
- Don't drink alcohol or smoke cigarettes.
- Relax quietly before bedtime with a warm bath.
- Reserve the bed for sleep and sex.
- Get out of bed if you're not sleepy. Do some light reading or listen to music until the sandman returns.

CHAPTER 21

Irritable bowel syndrome

What is irritable bowel syndrome? These muscle spasms in the stomach or intestines are also known as spastic colon, nervous bowel, or simply IBS. The cause is unknown, but stress and depression can aggravate it. It isn't life-threatening, but it can affect your quality of life.

Who gets it? About one in five American adults gets IBS. Women and children get it more often than men.

What are the symptoms?

- abdominal cramps and pain
- diarrhea
- constipation
- gas and bloating
- indigestion

Foods that fuel and foil flare-ups

Your best defense against the painful cramping, bloating, and other symptoms of irritable bowel syndrome (IBS) is a low-fat, high-fiber diet. But choosing the right foods can be tricky. Within these food groups are some that ease and others that bring on symptoms.

Find the best fats. Digesting fats can cause bloating and painful colon contractions. So go easy on red meats, which tend to have a lot of fat. On the other hand, fish like salmon and tuna – with omega-3 fatty acids – can ease an irritated bowel. Flaxseed oil, another good source of omega-3 fatty acids, also helps.

Cut back on most dairy. The extra fat found in regular dairy foods can trigger the symptoms of IBS. But after switching to skim milk and low-fat cheeses, you may still experience problems with lactose intolerance. This means you can't digest the sugar in milk and other dairy products.

Eating yogurt with live cultures, however, may make it easier to digest lactose.

Artichoke leaf, which is available in liquid or capsule form in health food stores, relieves symptoms of IBS. Make sure to talk to your doctor first if you're pregnant, have gallbladder disease, or take medication for high cholesterol.

Choose vegetables and fruits carefully. The fiber in plant foods helps move everything smoothly through your system. Fresh is best, as prepackaged foods tend to be harder to digest. If you haven't been eating a lot of fiber, add it gradually to cut down on gas.

You may need to pass on beans, broccoli, and cabbage, which can cause gas. Certain other fruits and vegetables, if eaten raw, may cause distress as well.

Drink plenty of the right liquids. Water helps ease the fiber through your system. Peppermint or chamomile tea can help, too, by soothing muscle spasms.

But carbonated beverages, caffeinated drinks of all kinds, and decaffeinated coffee may bring on gas pains.

Be selective about sweeteners. Sugar-free sweeteners, like sorbitol and mannitol, can give you gas. Sucrose, found naturally in fruits and honey, can also be a problem for some. But for those who can tolerate it, honey may ease constipation and clear up diarrhea associated with IBS.

Avoid fluffy foods. A main cause of gas is swallowed air, so go slow on milk shakes, whipped cream, and soufflés.

White bread, by the way, has more air — and less fiber — than whole wheat bread.

Healthy habits

Diet is just one strategy for eliminating the discomforts of irritable bowel syndrome. Here are some others.

- Eat slowly and chew well.
- Exercise to speed up digestion and move gas through your system.
- Get plenty of sleep.
- Breathe deeply and pratice relaxing to reduce stress.
- Avoid irritants like tobacco and alcohol.
- Talk to your doctor about taking antibiotics.

CHAPTER 22

Kidney stones

What are kidney stones? They are pebble-like crystals that form when certain chemicals build up in your urine.

Who gets them? One out of 10 people suffers a kidney stone in his lifetime. Men are more prone to them than women, but kidney problems and family history also put you at risk.

What are the symptoms?

- bloody, smelly, cloudy, or burning urine
- urge to urinate often
- stabbing, irregular pain in the back or side
- fever, chills, or weakness
- nausea or vomiting

Design your meals to avoid stones

Only certain foods contain the "fab four" of kidney stone prevention. They are the nutrients your kidneys require to stay healthy – magnesium, potassium, calcium, and vitamin B6.

The following meal plan teams these nutrients together with other kidney friendly food components. It's an example of how to make the fab four a regular part of your diet.

Breakfast:

- a bowl of oatmeal
- fresh raspberries

Whole grains, like those in hearty oatmeal, are super sources of magnesium. This multi-talented mineral helps your body

recycle oxalate, so the compound doesn't build up to dangerous levels in your urine.

Besides magnesium, oatmeal is tops in fiber, too. One cup can
have as many as 4 grams. Along with the fiber in fresh raspberries, this will put you well on your way to the daily fiber
requirement for people age 50 and over – 30 grams for men
and 21 grams for women. Research shows that even just 10 to
15 grams of fiber a day might help prevent kidney stones.

Lunch:

- a tossed salad with avocado slices

- a baked potato

- a glass of lemonade

The salad and the baked potato will boost your potassium
levels. This vital nutrient lowers the calcium levels in your
urine, which then lowers your risk of forming stones. Most
fruits and vegetables contain potassium, as do legumes, dairy
foods, and fish.

The steamy baked potato and avocado come with another
stone-stopping nutrient – vitamin B6. Just as magnesium does,
vitamin B6 helps your body maintain safe oxalate levels. Other
major sources are fortified cereals, bananas, and prunes.

For your beverage, enjoy refreshing lemonade. Its tartness
comes from citric acid, a substance that dissolves stones
before they grow painfully big. For homemade lemonade,
mix 4 ounces of lemon juice with two quarts of water and
sweeten lightly. This recipe seemed to do the trick in a recent
small study.

As for other citrus drinks, they can't compare with lemonade.
Orange juice has five times less citric acid than its popular
counterpart. And grapefruit juice, despite its citric acid, may
increase your odds of forming kidney stones.

Snack:

- low-fat yogurt
- dried fruit trail mix

Calcium from foods like yogurt may bind with the oxalate in your system and make it harmless. Besides yogurt, the mineral's sources include other low-fat dairy products, sardines, broccoli, black-eyed peas, and turnip greens.

You can tell kidney stones to take a hike with the magnesium you'll get from the dried fruit trail mix. Or snack on the mineral's other sources — seeds, legumes, artichokes, beet greens, and rice.

Dinner:

- a salmon filet
- black beans and rice
- wedge of honeydew melon

Your last meal of the day will round out your supply of potassium, magnesium, and vitamin B6. By this time, the fab four will be a big hit with your kidneys.

11 foods that aren't kind to your kidneys

You may have foods in your kitchen that contain oxalate, a natural plant chemical that's also a major ingredient in kidney stones. Though some may be your favorites, steer clear of them if you have a history of kidney stones. They include soy products, coffee, cola, spinach, beets, nuts, chocolate, tea, wheat bran, strawberries, and rhubarb.

Be wary of these popular myths

It bombards you every day from your newspapers, magazines, and neighbors – the latest, greatest health advice. But many times, following it may actually put you more at risk for health problems, including kidney stones.

Myth 1: A high-protein, low-carbohydrate diet is a healthy way to lose weight.

"This type of diet increases the propensity to develop kidney stones," says Dr. Chia-Ying Wang, a professor at the University of Texas Southwestern Medical Center. "People may lose weight on this diet, but this study shows that this is not a healthy way to lose weight."

Wang should know. She and her colleagues recently finished an eight-week study that showed how a high-protein diet could increase your kidney stone risk. First, these meal plans typically call for plenty of meat, which may cause your blood acid level to skyrocket.

Meanwhile, the diet may lower your urinary citrate levels by nearly 25 percent. Since citrate is a chemical that helps dissolve stones, this could be a disaster for your kidneys.

If you follow one of these popular plans, at least consider giving up some animal-based protein. Replace it with plant foods high in protein, like bulgur, barley, rice, and beans. Or better yet, talk with your doctor about a safer plan to lose weight.

Myth 2: Drinking eight glasses of water a day is an absolute must for everybody.

"After a 10-month search," Dr. Heinz Valtin reports, "I have not found a single scientific article that says we should drink eight glasses of water a day." This left Valtin, professor emeritus at Dartmouth Medical School, with a dramatic conclusion.

You don't need to drink eight 8-ounce glasses of water every day – if you're a healthy adult in a temperate climate.

However, if you're prone to kidney stones, this may not include you. "Most doctors probably recommend eight glasses of water for kidney stones," Valtin says.

You may even want to drink as much as three to four quarts of water a day – more if you exercise or the weather is hot. The increased fluid will dilute your urine and wash away stone-building chemicals like acid and oxalate before they build up.

And unlike what you might have heard, soda, coffee, tea, and other caffeinated beverages count toward your eight-a-day total, Valtin claims.

Of course, before you drink a gallon of any liquid, get your doctor's expert opinion. Drinking too much of anything – including water – can be harmful.

Myth 3: Kidney stone sufferers should avoid calcium because it's a major stone ingredient.

True, calcium is a common ingredient in kidney stones. Yet, surprisingly eating foods high in calcium seems to prevent stones. Confused? Scientists aren't.

They believe that dietary calcium binds with dietary oxalate while the two compounds are in your digestive system. Otherwise, they could become concentrated in your urine, crystallize, and grow into a stone.

So stock up on foods rich in calcium. These include low-fat dairy products, sardines, oysters, broccoli, black-eyed peas, peanuts, and turnip greens.

Be cautious with calcium supplements. Unlike food sources, this form of calcium might increase your risk of kidney stones.

Healthy habits

Once you have one kidney stone, you're more likely to have another. That's a good reason to follow these day-to-day suggestions to prevent them.

- Cut back on salty and sugary foods.

- Drink at least three to four quarts of fluids a day — more if you exercise or it's hot outside. Start when you wake up, and don't quit until your head hits the pillow.

- Get some protein by eating a variety of plant-based foods, like barley, bulgur, rice, oats, legumes, broccoli, and leafy greens, instead of red meat and poultry.

- Flip sides in bed so you don't sleep on the same one for too long.

CHAPTER 23

Macular degeneration

What is macular degeneration? Age-related macular degeneration (AMD) is a breakdown of the macula, the central part of the retina with your sharpest vision. It is irreversible and a leading cause of blindness.

Who gets it? AMD usually begins in the late 50s or 60s and is likely to occur in one third of people over age 75. High risk factors are smoking, light-colored eyes, long-time sun exposure, high blood pressure, heart disease, and family history of AMD or heart disease.

What are the symptoms?

- gradual blurring or blind spots in central field of vision
- printed words and fine details difficult to pick out, straight lines appear wavy, shapes distorted
- dimmed color vision

Slash AMD risk in half

You've probably encouraged your children to eat carrots to help their eyesight. If so, you were on the right track. That's because carrots are full of beta carotene, which converts to vitamin A – essential to good eyesight.

Studies have shown that people who eat more carotenoids like beta carotene have a 43 percent lower risk of developing age-related macular degeneration (AMD). But two other carotenoids may be even more important in avoiding AMD, says Barbara Gollman, food and nutrition consultant and author of *The Phytopia Cookbook: A world of plant-centered cuisine.*

"Lutein and zeaxanthin, pigments found in the retina, have the most scientific research behind them for keeping eyes healthy," she says. These two substances are highly concentrated in the part of the retina called the macula, which is the area affected by AMD.

Scientists are paying a lot more attention to lutein and zeaxanthin – sometimes called the "macular pigment" or MP – because they are the only carotenoids found within the retina. MP fights cell damage by filtering certain harmful light rays and as an antioxidant to fight free radicals.

Foods with a good supply of carotenoids can save your eyesight, no matter what your age. So fill your grocery cart with these foods and help reduce your risk of blindness in old age by nearly half.

Grab on to greens. Dark green leafy vegetables, like spinach, kale, collard, mustard and turnip greens, are the best foods to find lutein and zeaxanthin, according to Gollman. Broccoli and romaine lettuce are also good sources, she says.

Fresh kale has more lutein than any other food classified by the USDA. It also has more combined lutein and zeaxanthin. Raw spinach is next on the list, followed by fresh-cooked turnip and collard greens.

When selecting fresh spinach, kale, and other greens, look for crisp green leaves. Avoid leaves that are bruised, broken, wilted, moldy, or splotchy. Wash thoroughly to get rid of grit or sand.

Although raw greens have more nutrients, you'll absorb them better if you cook them. A study has shown that a little fat also helps with absorption, so you might try sauteing your greens lightly in olive oil to get the most carotenoids possible.

Get more MPs from red grapes. Red seedless grapes are high on the list of foods that contain both macular pigments. Try the Flame Seedless variety, a mildly sweet fruit with a touch of tartness and a crunchy bite.

They make a healthful between-meal snack. Store grapes in a plastic bag in the refrigerator for up to a week and make sure you rinse them well before popping them in your mouth.

Pick orange peppers. The richest source of zeaxanthin is the orange bell pepper. All sweet peppers are packed with nutrients, but more of the orange pepper's carotenoids are zeaxanthin than anything else. When selecting peppers, avoid those with poor color or bruises. Keep them refrigerated in a covered container or bag, and they'll also last up to a week.

Shop for cantaloupes. Like carrots, cantaloupes are rich in vitamin C and beta carotene. These all-star antioxidants help protect your retina from free radical damage and keep the blood vessels in your eye healthy. A small cantaloupe contains more than 180 mg of vitamin C. Eat one every day and you can reduce your chances of AMD by one-third.

Reconsider eggs. Perhaps a surprising source of lutein and zeaxanthin is the egg yolk. A study has shown that 89 percent of the carotenoids in egg yolks are lutein or zeaxanthin – a higher percentage than in any other food.

It's easy to overdo eggs, which are sometimes frowned on because they're high in cholesterol. Some studies suggest, however, that eggs help increase HDL cholesterol, which protects against atherosclerosis. So eating a few eggs each week may not be such a bad idea for both your heart and your eyes.

One way to keep your eyes healthy is to fix a colorful salad every day using a variety of these foods. You'll have something that looks good, tastes good, gives amazing strength to your retinas, and protects against the risk of AMD as you get older.

Recruit extra protection for your eyes

You need as many troops as you can muster in your battle against age-related macular degeneration. Carotenoids are a good front-line defense, but extra soldiers can further slow the advance of AMD's irreversible effects.

So what foods should you recruit?

In a nutshell, nuts are good. So are red grapes, cranberries, fruit peelings, mangoes, avocados, onions, beans, and tuna fish. These things aren't magic cures, but they are full of antioxidants that can make some of the risk disappear.

Find flavonoids in grapes. An occasional glass of red wine may help lower your risk of AMD. Researchers have found that grape skins contain flavonoids – powerful antioxidants that fight free radicals. Don't count on white wine, though, because white wine doesn't use grape skins. Beer is also not a good choice. It not only contains no grapes, it has been shown to increase your risk of AMD. If you don't drink alcohol, you can take advantage of the flavonoids in red seedless grapes and refreshing grape juice.

Discover the benefits of PCO. Another powerful set of bioflavonoids called procyanidolic oligomers (PCO) come from a certain kind of pine bark. PCO joins with vitamins C and E to get rid of the free radicals that cause so much damage to the center of your eyes. It also strengthens the capillaries in your eyes, which can weaken and rupture as you age.

> The herbal remedy ginkgo biloba is good for your eyes, too. It works as an antioxidant and widens, or dilates, your blood vessels.

PCO is also found inside grape seeds and is sold as pine bark (pycnogenol) or grape seed extract. You can get these antioxidants naturally, however, from grape skins, other citrus peels, apples, onions, blueberries, cranberries, and peanuts.

Think zinc for eye protection. Researchers noticed that low levels of zinc often went along with a higher risk of AMD. In their studies, they found that zinc actually helps other substances shield your eyes from AMD. People who took zinc along with vitamins C, E, and beta carotene were less likely to get AMD than those taking just the vitamins or zinc.

You usually get plenty of zinc from your regular diet, but sometimes young children, pregnant women and older people don't get enough. The best source is red meat, and seafood like oysters and crabmeat, but you can also get it from whole grains, yogurt, black beans, and lima beans.

Stick to foods for this important mineral because you could end up getting a dangerous amount from supplements. You should not use zinc supplements without talking with your doctor first.

Dig up some selenium. Another trace mineral, selenium, acts as an antioxidant but also works a lot like zinc — by improving the effect of vitamins E and C. Selenium comes from the soil so unprocessed foods are a good source for it. Go for Brazil nuts, grains, fresh vegetables, and also seafood.

A good selenium-filled lunch would be a cup of barley soup, a tuna fish sandwich made with whole grain bread, and a stalk of celery. As with zinc, it's better to get selenium from foods than from supplements. Too much of it is just as dangerous as not enough.

Go nuts for vitamin E. For a sunny outlook in preserving your eyesight, munch on a handful of sunflower seeds. Or try almonds or hazelnuts. You'll get a large load of vitamin E, one of several nutrients that work together to slow down the progress of AMD. A recent study showed that high doses of vitamins E, C, and beta carotene plus zinc lowered the risk of advanced AMD by 25 percent.

Your body absorbs natural vitamin E better than supplements, so along with nuts and seeds, focus on eating foods like sweet potatoes, avocados, or mangoes. Or try sprinkling some wheat germ on your breakfast cereal. All are good sources of this valuable antioxidant.

Brighten your sight with yellow lenses

Seeing the world through rose-colored glasses isn't as wonderful as you might think. If you have macular degeneration, lemon-colored lenses may be better, according to a small British study.

Researchers wanted to find out if tinted lenses helped people with AMD see better. Fifteen elderly subjects — 10 with AMD — wore special red, yellow, orange, and gray glasses for seven days.

Researchers discovered that yellow and orange lenses added brightness and that the gray lenses helped distinguish contrast when there was too much glare.

People in the early stages of AMD said the yellow lenses helped them see more distinctly and were best for overall improved vision. Yellow also scored high with non-AMD subjects, but red lenses seemed worse for both groups.

Keep your eyes fit with fish

Add your eyesight to the list of things you can save by watching your fat intake. Not only are obese men twice as likely to develop macular degeneration, but eating too much fat also increases your risk for this disease.

It's not just saturated fat you have to worry about, either. At least one study has shown that monounsaturated and polyunsaturated fats may harm your eyes just as much. Scientists think fat-clogged arteries around your eyes contribute to macular degeneration the way blockages in your chest can trigger a heart attack. The solution is to focus on eating certain types of fat and continue to cut back on the harmful ones.

Eat fatty fish. A Harvard study concludes that people who get their fat from fish – especially tuna – don't get AMD as much as those who eat other kinds of fat.

For several years, researchers at the Harvard School of Public Health followed 567 participants from the long-running Nurses' Health Study and the Health Professional Follow-up Study. They saw positive evidence that those who ate more animal and vegetable fat were more likely to get AMD. They also found that eating lots of fish may cut back on your chances of developing this disease.

The value of fish fat may come from an omega-3 fatty acid called docosahexaenoic acid (DHA) found in the retina of your eye. The study showed that the more DHA you have, the lower your risk of AMD. However, researchers found the same inverse relationship with fish in general so it's possible a combination of nutrients may be responsible for the protective effect.

In any case, eating fish seems to be a positive step for the health of your eyes. After tuna, your best choices are other cold-water fish like mackerel, salmon, and sardines. Non-fish foods with omega-3 fatty acids are walnuts, flaxseed, and wheat germ.

Substitute snack foods. You can get rid of unhealthy fats in your diet by rearranging some of your snack food choices. Try these ideas to have stronger eyes, better heart health, and left-over grocery money.

- Substitute popcorn for potato chips in front of the TV.

- Order a baked potato instead of french fries when you're at a restaurant. Just don't load up on butter, sour cream, cheese, and bacon bits in the process.

- Replace fried apple pies with just plain apples. Oranges, pears, and plums are also easy, tasty snacks.

- Nibble on grapes, raisins, or walnuts instead of candy bars and processed cookies and crackers.

Healthy habits

You can't control conditions like age, family history, and light-colored eyes that put you at risk for macular degeneration. But you can give yourself extra protection with these sight-saving strategies.

- **Stay away from smoke.** Whether it's your own or the second-hand variety, cigarette smoke promotes damaging free radicals. If you haven't already quit, right now is a good time.

- **Shade your eyes.** The sun's ultraviolet rays also create free radicals. Use sunglasses and a wide-brimmed hat or baseball cap.

- **Manage your weight.** Both too much and too little weight increases your risk for AMD. Learn your ideal weight and work to maintain it. This could cut your risk by 50 percent.

- **Take your medicine.** Statins, a group of anti-cholesterol drugs, seem to go along with a low rate of AMD. It could be their anti-cholesterol or antioxidant powers that protect your eyes. If you have a cholesterol problem, statins might provide a double benefit.

CHAPTER 24

Menopause

What is menopause? Menopause occurs when the ovaries stop producing eggs each month, hormone levels — especially estrogen — drop, and menstruation ends. It can happen all at once, if ovaries are surgically removed, or more gradually, over several years.

When does it occur? For half of all women, menopause takes place by age 50. It may happen earlier or later depending on your genes.

What are the symptoms? Before menstruation ends, you may have irregular periods that are very light or very heavy. Other symptoms include hot flashes, mood swings, indigestion, vaginal dryness, sleep loss, forgetfulness, weight gain, urinary tract infections, vaginal infections, and depression.

Avoid HRT with a natural food plan

Researchers recently stopped a large hormone replacement therapy (HRT) study because they were concerned about health risks. Five years into the study, they were startled to see a significant increase in invasive breast cancer as well as other health problems. Their research showed:

- a 26-percent rise in breast cancer

- 22 percent more cardiovascular disease

- a 29-percent increase in heart attacks

- a 41-percent jump in stroke

- twice the rate of blood clots

That translates into seven to eight more cancer or heart disease cases per 10,000 HRT users each year. That may not seem like a lot, but when you look at the population as a whole, it could mean thousands more health problems over time.

As a result, the Food and Drug Administration (FDA) now advises doctors to prescribe HRT only when benefits clearly outweigh health risks. The FDA says doctors should prescribe HRT just long enough for successful treatment – and at the lowest effective dose. What's more, women should consider other treatments for vaginal dryness and osteoporosis.

Reversing the long-held notion that HRT protects against heart disease, both the FDA and American Heart Association now warn against using hormone therapy to reduce the chances of heart problems.

So what can you do to balance your body chemistry during menopause? Some experts suggest a natural eating plan may help you survive menopause and control the related risks of heart disease, osteoporosis, and cancer. That means you should make a nutritious diet your first line of defense.

These expert tips will help you fill your body with vital nutrients that ease menopausal symptoms and fight serious disease.

- Focus on foods that come from plants. Many contain substances that may help regulate hormones.

- Pick foods that are fresh, unrefined, and unprocessed, emphasizing fruits and vegetables. Try locally grown produce for just-picked freshness.

- Choose more whole grains. Rich in hormone-regulators and nutrition, whole grains include oats, whole wheat, rye, millet, barley, and corn.

- Eat beans and peas for their hormone regulators. Chickpeas, lima beans, and kidney beans are good examples. To help you decide whether to eat soybeans and other soy foods, see *Be wise about soy* on page 198.

- Include extra-virgin olive oil in your diet.

- Eat cold-water, fatty fish rich in omega-3 oils. Salmon, mackerel, and albacore tuna are good examples.

- Replace refined white and brown sugar with raw honey and real maple syrup.

- Replace table salt with herbs and spices.

The following diet changes will help you avoid chemicals that may throw off your hormone balance and raise your odds of serious disease.

- Eat organic foods often. Avoid foods with additives, colorings, or preservatives.

- Snub hydrogenated oils, partially hydrogenated oils, and trans fatty acids, such as those in margarine. If a food includes a partially or fully hydrogenated oil in its label, try to find a substitute.

- Drink plenty of water, but filter it or use natural spring water. Unfiltered tap water is often contaminated with chemicals and bacteria.

- Eat meat sparingly. To start cutting back, eat smaller portions of beef, poultry, and pork.

- Limit alcohol to small amounts, and don't drink often.

- Don't drink diet soda and soft drinks. They are high in phosphorous, which can leech minerals from your bones. Plus the sugar and synthetic sweeteners they contain have their own negative effects.

- Give up caffeine as soon as possible. Look for more natural ways to boost your energy.

Remember, every time you add nutritional superstars to your diet or reject those that are bad for you, you rev up your body's defenses. A stronger body will go a long way toward protecting you against health risks and unpleasant menopausal symptoms.

Double your defense with diet

You haven't changed your diet at all, but suddenly you're gaining weight. If you're facing menopause, that may be the key to your problem. But don't worry – you can target your weight and your menopause symptoms at the same time by following these nutrition tips.

Learn the latest. A small study found that women are more likely to store fat in the stomach and buttock areas after menopause because their metabolism changes during the "change of life." But don't give up hope. By reducing your total calories as you near menopause, you'll help limit weight gain, says the study's author, Dr. Cynthia Ferrara, a professor in the University of Maryland School of Medicine. Cutting calories may also cut the fat you store at the waist, she adds.

"The best advice for a woman nearing or experiencing the menopause transition would be to try to prevent some of the increases in body weight through diet and regular exercise," she says.

Examine your diet. Lifestyle changes – such as a high-fiber, low-fat diet rich in antioxidants – may help lower menopause risks and symptoms, suggests the American Academy of Family Physicians. Fruits, cereals, and vegetables fit the bill perfectly. A 10-year study found that people who ate at least 19 servings of vegetables a week were less likely to add weight at the waist compared to those who ate relatively few servings.

Try eating more low-calorie cereals and fruits and vegetables, especially the ones packed with nutrients that could soothe menopause symptoms and lower related risks, such as osteoporosis and heart disease.

Turn on to turnip greens. If you ever sit down to a "meat and three" meal in the southeastern United States, don't be surprised to see turnip greens on your plate. This old "Dixie" favorite may become a favorite of yours when you learn what its calcium can do. Even though one study suggests bone loss can reach 1 percent per year during menopause, getting more calcium may fight bone loss. What's more, some nutritionists say calcium might help hot flashes, too.

Get up to 249 milligrams (mg) of calcium from a cup of turnip greens for just 29 calories. Try kale or Chinese cabbage (bok choy) for more calorie-scrimping calcium. But what if you crave something sweet? Check the labels of fortified orange juices for high calcium and a "no added sugar" claim. One study found that drinking a cup of orange juice 30 minutes before a meal could help you feel more full and eat fewer calories – perhaps 300 fewer.

Select the right cereal. You need vitamin D to protect your bones because it plays an important role in how much calcium your bones actually absorb. Pour some low-fat or nonfat milk on vitamin-D-fortified cereal for a double dose of protection. Check the labels to figure out which cereal has the most vitamin D and the least amount of calories.

Bring on the broccoli. Little trees bring lots of E that might ease menopause. Vitamin E may sap hot flashes and help your skin stay softer. If you drink lots of water while loading up on E, you might ease vaginal dryness.

Cook a cup of frozen broccoli for a little over 3 mg of vitamin E, about 20 percent of the recommended dietary allowance. Low-calorie turnip greens and mustard greens also pack in vitamin E. For a delicious and healthy treat, try fresh peaches, almonds, or sunflower seeds.

So fill your meals with low-calorie fruits and veggies. With this fat-fighting arsenal of nutrition, you can minimize menopause symptoms now while building a healthier body for the years to come.

Be wise about soy

When menopause steals your estrogen, replace it with plant sources. Eating plant foods with phytoestrogens can give you some of the protective benefits of estrogen. Good sources include oats, wheat, corn, apples, almonds, cashews, and peanuts.

A specific kind of phytoestrogen, called isoflavones, are found mostly in soy-based foods like soybeans, tofu, miso, and soy nuts. Asian women who eat one type of soy food every day report very few hot flashes and mood swings during menopause. This could mean they're getting some estrogen from their diet.

Unfortunately, experts have concerns. Although some research shows soy might help your heart and prevent osteoporosis, other studies suggest it makes your brain age faster. Various health experts think the more soy you eat, the greater your risk of developing senility.

Just to be on the safe side, talk with your doctor about the pros and cons of eating soy during menopause.

Master menopause with herbs

Are you having a hard time deciding whether to use herbs for menopause symptoms? Some people are enthusiastic about herbs while others think they're dangerous. Here's what you need to know about the most commonly recommended herbs for menopause.

Get help from black cohosh. The German equivalent of the Food and Drug Administration approved black cohosh for menopause symptoms years ago. What's more, a recent German study found that black cohosh taken twice a day may improve physical and emotional menopause symptoms. Other studies suggest that black cohosh may ease hot flashes, but relief could take four to six weeks.

Hot flashes are a problem for breast cancer survivors, especially those on tamoxifen. A recent study discovered that two months of daily black cohosh may not help hot flashes in breast cancer survivors, but it might ease sweating.

Keep in mind that black cohosh may give some women an upset stomach. Large doses may even cause nausea and dizziness. Until long-term safety studies can be done, don't take black cohosh for more than six months.

Vanquish insomnia with valerian. A recent German study found that valerian extract may relieve mild insomnia. In earlier studies, valerian users reported that they got to sleep faster and slept better.

In the United States, capsules containing 400 to 530 milligrams (mg) of whole ground valerian root are generally taken 30 to 60 minutes before bedtime. You may also find capsules of a root extract, liquid extracts, and tinctures.

If you prefer a tea, use one teaspoon of dried valerian root per cup. Valerian is sometimes used to treat uterine contractions, so if you are pregnant, check with your doctor before using this herb.

Review red clover. A small Dutch study reported over 40 percent fewer hot flashes with a daily red clover supplement containing 80 mg of isoflavones. On the other hand, two small clinical trials in Australia found no benefit from red clover. But red clover may affect more than just menopause.

Some experts think red clover may lower the higher cardiovascular risk that follows menopause. Although studies suggest red clover does not lower cholesterol, it may help your blood vessels stretch more easily. No one knows whether that means a lower risk of death from heart disease, but more flexible arteries may shrink the risk of heart trouble.

Red clover contains several isoflavones including genistein and daidzein. Initial research studies suggest that genistein could be connected to breast cancer tumor growth, senility, brain aging, and slowed thyroid activity. More research is needed to confirm or disprove these findings.

The University of Pittsburgh Cancer Institute recently discovered that red clover may also have high estrogenic activity – a possible risk for breast cancer. If your family history or personal history includes breast cancer, don't try red clover.

Stay dry with evening primrose oil. Studies have found that evening primrose oil might reduce night sweats although it does not seem to control hot flashes. No one knows whether it is safe to use for long periods, so if you try this herb, just take it for a short time to see if it helps. Never take evening primrose oil with nonsteroidal anti-inflammatory drugs (NSAIDs) or anticonvulsant drugs.

Don't single out dong quai. Dong quai is an ancient Chinese remedy for feminine complaints. Yet a six-month study found that dong quai alone may not help hot flashes or night sweats. On the other hand, Chinese herbalists argue that dong quai is not supposed to work alone. They say it must be part of a combination of herbs because the herbs must work together to be effective. Although herbal combinations are on the market, none have been tested.

Dong quai may cause bleeding in some people, especially those taking warfarin. It also makes your skin sensitive, so anyone using this herb should stay out of the sun.

The best thing to do is to ask your doctor before trying herbs. You'll enjoy herbal benefits even more when you know they're safe to take.

Healthy habits

Some women simply breeze through menopause. If you're not one of them, try these ideas to help control your symptoms and make life a little easier.

- Regular exercise fights weight gain, insomnia, and hot flashes. It also cuts your risk of heart disease and osteoporosis. Try to include both aerobic exercise, like brisk walking, swimming, or bicycling, and some type of resistance exercise like weight training or gardening. Don't forget to stretch before and after.

- If you already exercise, don't overdo it. Replace long heavy workouts with lighter workouts done more often.

- Give up smoking, and you may have fewer hot flashes.

- To help take the heat out of those "power surges," take cool baths and showers.

- When a hot flash starts, breathe in slowly through your nose so your abdomen expands. When your abdomen feels full, let the air out slowly through your nose.

CHAPTER 25 *Muscle cramps*

What are muscle cramps? These are painful, uncontrollable spasms or tightening in a muscle that can last for minutes, hours, or days. Sometimes the muscle can harden or twitch. Cramps most often occur in the thigh, calf, or foot.

Who gets them? Nighttime calf cramps are common among seniors. If you over-exercise, are dehydrated, have a nutrient imbalance, take certain medications, suffer from thyroid or nerve disorders or cardiovascular disease, or are a woman, you are more at risk for muscle cramps.

What are the symptoms?

- a tight, knotted, or hard feeling in a muscle
- sudden shooting pain
- soreness, general weakness, and fatigue

Get a leg up on muscle cramps

Once upon a time, cramp sufferers had only one remedy — quinine tablets. But these can be toxic in large doses. Today, experts know you don't need to put your body at risk to nip the pain of cramps. Rely on these all natural, safe alternatives instead.

Vanquish cramps with vitamin E. Just 400 international units (IU) of vitamin E every night for two months meant fewer muscle cramps for those involved in a controlled study.

Not only that, but the cramps they did have were less severe than usual. And when this antioxidant went head-to-head with quinine, it proved just as potent — without side effects.

This study had its limitations, however. Two months is a relatively short time to reach a positive conclusion, and all of the people had muscle cramps for the same reason – as a side effect of dialysis. Still, the researchers believe vitamin E is a good treatment for muscle cramps in general.

Although the study used supplements, you can benefit from eating food sources of vitamin E, like wheat germ, vegetable oils, and sunflower seeds.

> **When a muscle cramp hits, lower the affected limb below the rest of your body, put some heat on the muscle, or sit, stretch, and flex it.**

Wash them out with water. Dehydration is one of the most common causes of muscle cramps. Thankfully, it's also one of the easiest to fix. Drink eight 8-ounce glasses of water a day, especially when you're active or it's hot outside.

Pounce on pain with potassium. Your muscles demand a daily supply of this essential mineral to work properly. They'll protest and knot up if your body has an imbalance. Keep them happy instead with top potassium providers like beans, dates, raisins, spinach, bananas, and canned tomato products.

Soothe your muscles with magnesium. Just like potassium, magnesium is necessary for muscle health. This mineral helps to control how well muscles flex and relax. So a magnesium deficiency could be the secret cause of your muscle cramps and tiredness. For foods that can cure you, try dark leafy greens, nuts, legumes, and whole grains.

Calm cramps with calcium. The same mineral that keeps your bones strong keeps your muscles moving properly. Eat low-fat dairy foods, sardines, legumes, and other sources of calcium.

Stop soreness with vitamin C. If you're over 55, you have two reasons to take this potent vitamin – it strengthens muscles by repairing them and it powers up your immune system. No wonder some experts recommend taking a 500-milligram supplement of vitamin C before exercise.

Get this nutrient from natural sources such as strawberries, citrus fruit, broccoli, brussels sprouts, and sweet peppers.

Lighten the ache with leucine. This protein building block, also called an amino acid, repairs damaged muscles. That makes it excellent for easing the ache after a tough tennis match or long round of golf. For a dose of leucine, snack on a lean lunch meat like turkey, or a low-fat dairy food following your workout. Then wash it down with a carbohydrate-rich beverage, like juice or a sports drink.

Stop 'stitches' in their tracks

A muscle spasm can come on fast, but these three down-home cures fix them even faster.

Pickle juice. It's purely a home remedy, with no scientific backing, but many athletes, coaches, and trainers swear by it. Drink 2 ounces of this quirky cramp cure about an hour before exercising. For night cramps, sauerkraut may have the same effect. If you're on a salt-restricted diet, however, check with your doctor first.

Tonic water. Tonic contains enough quinine to fight cramps, but not enough to be harmful. Drink 8 ounces – and no more – before bedtime. Mix in some fruit juice to help cut the bitterness.

Mustard. Carry packets of this condiment with you whenever you exercise, advise physical trainers at the University of Alabama. Wash one down with water when muscle cramps hit. Then follow with another packet and water every two minutes until the spasms stop. Once again, be careful if you're salt sensitive.

Take 'heart' in the battle against leg cramps

Sometimes just a walk to the mailbox can cause your calves to clench. And a trip through the grocery store often means painful leg cramps. If this sounds familiar, you may have intermittent claudication.

This condition occurs when the blood vessels in your legs get clogged with cholesterol. Your muscles can't get enough oxygen-rich blood, so they ache during any kind of activity. The latest scientific evidence offers the most unlikely cure — exercise.

"Studies show that patients who exercise three or more times a week for at least three months have substantial increases in the distance they can walk without painful symptoms," announces Kerry J. Stewart, director of clinical exercise physiology at Johns Hopkins and lead researcher in the latest study. Your muscles seem to use even a limited blood supply more effectively after a good work out. Not to mention, exercise is good for your cardiovascular system in general.

To test this theory yourself, take a walk outside or on a treadmill. When your legs begin to hurt, fight through it and continue walking for several more minutes. Then stop. "After a few minutes of rest, the walking should be resumed," instructs Stewart, "and this cycle should be repeated until the person can walk for 50 minutes."

In addition to exercise, improve your circulation with these foods and herbal supplements.

Revive your arteries with grape juice. New research suggests your damaged blood vessels have hope – grape juice. This natural drink may make them more elastic and your blood less sticky. Experts believe antioxidants called flavonoids explain grape juice's healing powers.

It may, however, take a hearty amount of juice to get the same results as in the study. A 150-pound person, for instance, must drink 12 to 23 ounces of grape juice a day – that amount would fill one to two soda cans.

Remember that one cup of commercial unsweetened grape juice has 154 calories. So if you're watching your weight, drink the juice but cut out another snack.

Tame poor circulation with tea. The latest findings from Australia suggest that tea – black, oolong, or green – lowers the amount of a protein called P-selectin in your blood. The researchers believe P-selectin makes your blood clump together. So less is better for you and your heart.

Get going with ginkgo biloba. This ancient Chinese remedy works like aspirin to thin your blood and improve circulation to your legs. No wonder people say they can walk farther after taking ginkgo. Experts recommend 120 to 160 milligrams per day with meals.

Before taking ginkgo supplements, make sure yours is made from the plant's leaves and not the seeds, which could be harmful. Also, don't take it without your doctor's approval if you're already on aspirin or warfarin.

Crack cramps with nuts. Those suffering from intermittent claudication tend to be deficient in vitamin E. This makes sense, since the antioxidant is important for smooth blood flow. Nuts are one of the best natural sources of this nutrient, along with sunflower seeds, wheat germ, vegetable oils, and green leafy vegetables.

Beat leg pain with bulbs. Garlic and onions are cousins in the same plant family tree, and they inherited the same super benefits. Their health punch comes from special sulfate compounds, which make your blood less sticky. These compounds also give the bulbs their flavorful bite. So onions most likely to make you cry — yellow and red varieties — have the most blood-thinning powers. As for garlic, one bulb a day may do the trick. Once again, talk first with your doctor if you're on blood-thinning medication.

Healthy habits

You can take control over most kinds of muscle cramps by following these tips.

- Eat a well-rounded diet to keep your heart and muscles strong and your weight steady.

- Prevent muscle strain by clearing stairways, halls, and all walking space of clutter. When outdoors, watch for ice patches, water spills, debris, and anything else that may cause you to trip or fall.

- Wear proper-fitting shoes. Replace old ones as soon as the tread wears out or the heel becomes uneven.

- Get the green light from your doctor before you leap into a new sport, exercise, or physical activity.

- Warm up before exercise and stretch regularly.

- Hold off on exercise when you're tired or in pain.

- Stick to flat surfaces when you run, walk, or jog.

- Prop up your feet with a pillow if you frequently get leg cramps at night. Or dangle them off the bed's edge while lying facedown. This keeps you from flexing your feet and triggering a cramp.

CHAPTER 26

Nausea & vomiting

What is nausea and vomiting? Nausea is an uneasy feeling in your stomach. It sometimes leads to vomiting, which ejects your stomach's contents through your mouth.

Who gets it? Anybody can. But you are more prone to nausea and vomiting if you suffer from motion sickness, food poisoning, an infection or illness, vertigo, or food intolerances. Certain medications can also trigger it.

What are the symptoms?

- fever, sweats, chills, weakness, and unnatural paleness
- abdominal cramps or dry heaves
- inability to hold down solids or liquids
- unusual amount of saliva

Flavor your food with soothing spices

You know the question that comes to mind when salsa sets off a four-alarm fire in your mouth. How can people eat this stuff and like it? Here's the answer – it stops them from getting sick.

According to an eye-opening study, our ancestors began eating spices because they prevent food poisoning. Spices wipe out the bugs that cause it.

"We believe the ultimate reason for using spices is to kill food-borne bacteria and fungi," reports Dr. Paul W. Sherman, lead author of the study and Cornell University biology professor.

This explains why dishes from tropical places like Mexico and Thailand are loaded with spice. They need more protection there since food spoils more quickly in the heat. "People who enjoyed food with antibacterial spices probably were healthier, especially in hot climates," says Sherman.

No matter where you live, add spices and condiments to your food to save yourself from a bout of nausea and vomiting. Everyday flavor-savers like garlic, onion, allspice, and oregano tested best in the study. They killed 100 percent of all bacteria. Thyme, tarragon, cumin, and cinnamon weren't far behind on the list. The following spices, however, go beyond just eliminating bacteria.

Halt nausea with jalapenos. Believe it or not, hot peppers could rescue you if you get an upset stomach when you eat. People who took red pepper before meals suffered nearly two-thirds less nausea, bloating, and stomach pain in a small but significant study from Italy. Red pepper's active ingredient, capsaicin, seems to numb the stomach nerves that send pain signals to your brain.

In the study, they used a capsule form of red pepper, but you can achieve the same effect by eating three spicy meals. Talk with your doctor before heating up your diet, though. Capsaicin is a powerful compound and can bother stomachs, too.

Make ginger your trump card against cancer, arthritis, heart disease, and other ailments. According to research, ginger has one of the highest antioxidant loads in the plant kingdom.

Get results with ginger. Ginger has proven itself in study after study. It has cut off queasiness brought on by everything from motion sickness to chemotherapy to surgery.

But it's probably most famous for fighting travel sickness. For your next trip, buy candied ginger at the supermarket or health food store. Eat two pieces — each roughly 1 inch by one-quarter inch thick — an hour before your departure. Then take the same amount every four hours during the voyage. If you have ginger capsules, two 500-milligram pills is about the same dose.

Ginger is also recommended for nausea caused by indigestion. Chop up a 1-inch piece of fresh ginger and boil it in hot water for 10 minutes to make a stomach-soothing tea.

Tame sickness with turmeric. If heavy meals knock you down for the count with nausea, turmeric could lift you off the mat. This spice encourages your body to produce bile, which helps you digest fat.

The German Commission E, the world-famous herbal authority, recommends taking as much as half a teaspoon a day to overcome an upset stomach. Sprinkle it into your own stir fries or have a curry dish when you dine at an Asian restaurant. Turmeric is a big part of curry sauces.

Soothe your stomach with peppermint. A folk medicine backed by modern research, peppermint packs a one-two punch against stomach sickness. Like all of the plants in Sherman's study, peppermint kills bacteria. On top of that, it calms the muscles of your digestive tract.

To brew a delicious tea, pour 5 ounces of hot water over two teaspoons of peppermint leaves. Let it steep for 10 minutes. Make sure to check with your doctor first if you have liver or gallbladder disease.

Vanquish vomiting with chamomile. Chamomile may not make a good condiment, but it's sure worth trying on its own. The flower could prevent vomiting by calming spasms in your digestive system.

Like other plants on this list, chamomile is a treasure as a tea. Soak its leaves for 10 to 15 minutes in hot water in a covered container. Then strain and drink. If you have pollen allergies, however, be careful. You may also be allergic to chamomile.

Before you know it, you'll be a spice aficionado who's able to handle white-hot curries and sizzling salsas. And your stomach will thank you for it.

Foil a fatal side effect

Dehydration is one of the greatest dangers of being sick. Because of vomiting, sweating, and diarrhea, your body gets short on water and essential minerals like potassium and sodium. It's key to stop dehydration before it sets in.

Replenish fluids. Store-bought rehydration drinks, like Pedialyte, are specially formulated to prevent dehydration. Remember to sip these drinks slowly and often during your bout of sickness.

Make your own. You can also use this homemade rehydration beverage. Mix eight teaspoons of table sugar, half a teaspoon of salt, half a teaspoon of baking soda, and one-third of a teaspoon of potassium chloride into one liter of water.

See the signs. Untreated, dehydration leads to seizures, brain damage, and death. So watch for symptoms like sunken eyes; dry, sticky mouth; decreased urine; and deep, rapid breathing. Also, you can test your skin's elasticity by pinching your arm. You could be dehydrated if the skin slowly returns to place.

Rush to your doctor if you suspect you're dehydrated, especially if your vomiting lasts for more than 24 hours.

Settle your stomach in 3 steps

Food may seem like the last thing you want when you're sick, but the right kind can help baby your belly back to health.

Lead off with liquids. If you're nauseous and want to prevent vomiting, sip on something cool and sweet, like soda, juice, or a popsicle. Grapefruit and orange juice, though, are off limits because they're so acidic.

Liquids are also essential after you've been sick. Take in as many as possible without making yourself nauseous again. Try clear fluids like water, ginger ale, juice, and sports drinks. Broth, tea, cola, and light soups are kind to your stomach, too.

Regain balance with bland foods. Move on to solid foods when your vomiting spell passes. Start slow with small but frequent portions. Stick with starchy foods, such as crackers, dry toast, or cooked cereal. Stay away from strong-tasting or strong-smelling foods, as well as fried, greasy, or sweet foods. Don't mix hot and cold dishes.

Be a BRAT to your stomach. The BRAT eating plan is your final stop before returning to your normal diet. BRAT stands for bananas, rice, applesauce, and toast. These four nutritious foods are especially gentle on a stomach getting over food poisoning, but they're tender to any kind of upset stomach.

You'll be back to your old self in no time if you ease your way through this simple three-step plan.

Know when nausea means business

For one out of six seniors in a new study by Dr. John Canto, nausea was a symptom of angina. This dangerous condition occurs when your heart doesn't get enough oxygen. Most people think of chest pain as the only sign of angina, but nausea can also signal that you're one step away from a heart attack.

Nausea may point to other serious problems, including:

- kidney or liver disease
- brain tumors and central nervous system problems

- cancer

- head injury

- infections like encephalitis, appendicitis, or meningitis

- intestinal blockage

- migraine

- heatstroke

- overdose of zinc, magnesium, and other minerals

- anxiety

If you suffer from one of these conditions, you may also have vomit that's bloody or looks like coffee grounds. Or you may have a fever of 101 degrees Fahrenheit or higher, diarrhea, rapid breathing or pulse, severe abdominal pain, confusion, agonizing headache, stiff neck, or severe fatigue. Get to your doctor on the double if you notice any of these symptoms.

Healthy habits

These simple precautions can be the difference between a happy stomach and one that's turned upside down.

- Rinse produce before eating it. Pull off its outer leaves and husks and brush the skin if needed.

- Wash your hands before and after touching produce and raw meat.

- Don't buy bruised or damaged-looking produce.

- Store your groceries in the refrigerator as soon as possible after shopping.

- Sanitize cutting surfaces with hot water and soap or a 3-percent hydrogen peroxide solution.

- Avoid raw shellfish, unpasteurized juices and milk, and raw cookie dough.

- Defrost meat, poultry, and fish in your refrigerator or microwave, not at room temperature. Marinate food in the refrigerator, too.

- Separate raw meats from other foods.

- Set your refrigerator at 41 degrees Fahrenheit or less and your freezer at zero degrees.

- Throw away food that's been sitting out for more than two hours, including sliced produce.

- Eat only bland, starchy foods before a trip if you get motion sickness. Don't smoke or drink beforehand.

- Face front when traveling. Don't look out side windows.

CHAPTER 27 *Osteoarthritis*

What is osteoarthritis? Osteoarthritis (OA) is a joint disease where your cartilage – the spongy tissue that cushions your joints – gradually wears away, and your bones rub together. OA can develop in any joint, but especially in your hands, knees, hips, and back.

Who gets it? Over 20 million people in the United States have OA. The wear and tear of life contributes to OA, but overweight people, older women, and people with joint injuries are most at risk for this disease.

What are the symptoms?

- morning joint stiffness
- painful, swollen, tender joints
- joints that crack often

Wipe out OA with these vital nutrients

Fed up with arthritis? Then eat to end your pain. Pain-fighting nutrients found in many foods work with your body to ease inflammation and repair damaged joints.

Naturopathic doctors – who specialize in natural treatments like nutrition and exercise – have long known this. Ron Hobbs, a naturopathic doctor and professor at Bastyr University, agrees. "Nutrition is key."

In OA, cartilage breaks down faster than your body can rebuild it, so you need to eat plenty of joint-strengthening foods to fight back. "If you're not eating the nutrients, they're not in your blood," Hobbs warns, and your cartilage won't get what it needs to regrow. "You've got to have these nutrients on board."

Osteoarthritis, severe joint discomfort, bone deformities, back pain, and rheumatism – you can discover the secrets to restoring what has been damaged by topping your plate with these healing nutrients.

Wash away OA with water. The water in your joints acts like oil in a car engine – run low on it, and the parts start to grind together and wear down. Water even carries nutrients from your blood to your cartilage. No matter how healthy your diet, you still need this fluid to reap the benefits.

How much should a person drink each day? In Hobbs' opinion, "Generally more than they do." Since cartilage is made up mostly of water, your joints are especially at risk for dehydration. New research shows that not everyone needs eight glasses of water a day. Instead, Hobbs recommends you drink enough to go to the bathroom regularly, but not too often. How much that takes will depend on your body and your lifestyle.

Fight back with phytochemicals. Researchers at the University of North Carolina at Chapel Hill discovered that certain phytochemicals – nutrients naturally found in plants – lowered some people's risk for knee OA by 30 to 40 percent. The fantastic phytochemicals in this study? Vitamin E, lutein, and lycopene, among others. Hobbs isn't surprised. "They're good for the plant, and they're also good for the human being."

> **Choose tomato products, like tomato sauce and tomato paste, over raw tomatoes to get the most lycopene. Then add a little olive or canola oil to help your body absorb this phytochemical.**

Colorful fruits and vegetables are often rich in phytochemicals. Spinach, zucchini, and red seedless grapes are great sources of lutein, while red fruits like tomatoes, papaya, pink grapefruit, and watermelon pack loads of lycopene. To get your fill of vitamin E, look to olive and canola oils, as well as nuts, seeds, and wheat germ.

Dive in with D. By now you know you can help stop OA with antioxidants. But ordinary sunshine? Like the miracle it is, your skin turns sunlight into vitamin D, a nutrient that's "turning out to be incredibly important, especially for elders," says Hobbs.

This vitamin protects your cartilage and bones and helps your body absorb calcium, a mineral essential to building strong joints. Too little vitamin D in your diet raises your risk for OA, particularly in the hips.

Filling your quota of vitamin D could be as easy as spending five minutes in the sun two or three days a week, nine months a year. If you have dark skin or live in a colder climate, look to low-fat dairy products, eggs, and seafood such as shrimp, salmon, or tuna for an extra dose of vitamin D.

Sing the praises of C. Without this vitamin, your joints can weaken three times faster than normal. Your body needs vitamin C to make collagen, an essential part of bones, cartilage, muscles, and tendons.

> Scurvy was one of the first diseases linked to poor diet. The nutrient used to treat it, vitamin C, was originally called ascorbic acid, Latin for "without scurvy."

But this powerful antioxidant may also protect your joints. In one study, people with knee OA who ate a diet high in vitamin C felt their pain ease, while those who got less vitamin C saw their arthritis worsen faster.

Your body can't make this vitamin, so be sure to get plenty in your diet. Fruits and vegetables like oranges, strawberries, broccoli, and red peppers are treasure troves of vitamin C.

Bring on the boron. Does a tasty snack of apples, peanut butter, and raisins sound good to you? Then good news – it could help prevent arthritis! All three foods are bursting with boron, a mineral that plants absorb from the soil.

Most people in modern countries eat only about 1 to 2 milli-grams (mg) of boron each day. But nutrition experts believe get-ting between 3 and 10 mg a day could help prevent arthritis and even ease joint pain, swelling, and stiffness. Look for other foods high in boron such as leafy vegetables, nuts, and non-citrus fruits like pears and prunes.

Manage your manganese. This mineral helps your body build strong joints. Being deficient in it can cause a disease similar to osteoarthritis. Hobbs believes most modern diets don't contain enough manganese. Indeed, people who eat only refined wheats, like white bread, get half as much manganese as those who eat whole grains. Other foods including pineapple, black-berries, legumes, sweet potato, and nuts can help you meet your manganese needs.

While many of these nutrients are sold as supplements, whole foods are still the safest way to put them to work in your joints. Talk with your doctor if you're considering supplements, and be sure to discuss any diet changes as well. Your doctor can help you make these decisions and follow your progress.

New diet promises self-healing

A new diet claims to attack arthritis where it hurts the most, in your inflamed joints. In their popular book *Arthritis Survival*, osteopathic doctor Robert Ivker and naturopathic doc-tor Todd Nelson present the New Life Eating Plan as part of their mind, body, and spiritual treatment program for relieving the pain of osteoarthritis.

According to the authors, food allergies as well as acid and minerals that build up in your joints can aggravate inflamma-tion. Foods like dairy products, oranges, wheat, peanuts, red meat and poultry, and plants in the nightshade family, toma-toes, potatoes, peppers, and eggplant, are common culprits.

Under the New Life Eating Plan, you would cut these inflammatory foods out of your diet for at least three weeks, then add them back in one at a time and watch how your body reacts. If your arthritis flares up after eating a certain food, it could be the cause.

Read Ivker's and Nelson's *Arthritis Survival* for more details about this plan, but discuss any new diet with your doctor before changing your eating habits.

Discover natural alternatives to NSAIDs

Aspirin and ibuprofen may ease your arthritis pain, but they can also cause ulcers and damage your cartilage even more.

Over half the people who regularly take NSAIDs for arthritis develop bleeding in their stomach or intestines. NSAIDs may even damage weakened joints by speeding up the loss of cartilage, or slowing the repair of damaged cartilage.

Some proven natural remedies may work just as well, and without the severe side effects. But drug companies don't want you to know that. Nonsteroidal anti-inflammatory drugs (NSAIDs), such as aspirin, ibuprofen, and naproxen, are big business. They're among the most common medicines for treating OA.

Before you trade arthritis pain for more serious problems, get the facts about nutritional alternatives for managing your pain.

Spice up your life. Ginger and turmeric, the main ingredient in curry, are homegrown hits for relieving inflamed joints. The key is curcumin, a phytochemical found in both spices that reduces inflammation. Studies show it may even work as well as NSAIDs and with fewer side effects. Spice up your stir-fry with a sprinkle of ground curry, or brew a spot of ginger tea to baby your joints.

The Chinese have used ginger as a seasoning and a medicine for 2,500 years. It's not a root. It's a rhizome, part of the stem that grows underground.

Discuss these remedies with your doctor before going gung-ho with spices. Large doses of ginger may irritate your stomach, and both ginger and turmeric can enhance the effects of blood-thinning medications, like aspirin and warfarin.

Boost your B's. Simply getting more B vitamins in your diet could soothe your swollen joints. In a Missouri study, people with arthritis in their hands took 6,400 micrograms (mcg) of folic acid (B9) along with 20 mcg of cobalamin (B12) every day. They soon had fewer sore joints and as much gripping power as people who took NSAIDs.

You can't get the amount of B vitamins used in this study just from food, so talk with your doctor about taking supplements if you think more B vitamins might work for you.

If you want to get more B vitamins from food, eat dark leafy greens, legumes, and fortified cereals. They are full of folic acid. Fish, eggs, meat, and dairy foods carry loads of vitamin B12.

Add a little E. The powerful antioxidant vitamin E may ease inflammation and slow down the progress of OA. Half the people in a recent study felt less pain while getting 600 mg of this vitamin a day over the course of 10 days.

People in this study beefed up their vitamin E intake with supplements. However, this vitamin can affect how your blood clots. Play it safe by avoiding large doses of vitamin E supplements while you are taking blood-thinning medications. Vitamin E is easily found in wholesome foods, like wheat germ, sunflower seeds, and canola oil.

Reel in relief. Fishermen are full of tall tales, but one may be true. In a new lab study, cod liver oil slowed the destruction of cartilage and reduced pain and inflammation. That's nothing new to Ron Hobbs, a naturopathic doctor and professor at Bastyr University in Washington state.

Hobbs and other experts attribute the fish oil's healing powers to its vast store of omega-3 polyunsaturated fatty acids (PUFAs). If he could do only one thing for people besides urge them to exercise, says Hobbs, he would "make sure they got more omega-3 in their diet."

Be warned that fish oil supplements may contain toxins from the fish's food and water, although some experts say the risk is slim. Supplements can also interfere with certain medications. Discuss the pro's and con's with your doctor before dishing out the cod liver oil.

You could also skip the supplements and head for the source. Fatty fish, such as salmon, mackerel, albacore tuna, and sardines, are teeming with omega-3, while wheat germ, walnuts, and dark green leafy vegetables pack their own PUFA punch.

That said, sometimes NSAIDs really are the best medicine. Hobbs agrees that "anti-inflammatories have their place."

The trick is not to rely on NSAIDs alone to treat your OA. "Nonsteroidal anti-inflammatory drugs can be a short-term stopgap" to reduce out-of-control inflammation, says Hobbs, "but if you just keep taking the NSAIDs, and you don't deal with the cause, then you're not doing good medicine."

Heating vegetable oils to high temperatures destroys their vitamin E. Use them 'raw' as a dressing on salads or cooked vegetables to get the most vitamin E.

Instead, try a well-rounded approach that involves good nutrition, moderate exercise, and periods of rest. Be sure to discuss the options with your doctor. She can help you develop a game plan and stick with it.

Rub on rapid relief

Tired of popping pills for your arthritis pain? Smooth on soothing creams instead. Certain topical creams contain natural ingredients to ease achy joints.

Apply the arnica. Ointments made from the arnica plant reduce inflammation and soothe mild aches and pains. Arnica can be poisonous if swallowed, so only use it externally. Stop using the cream if you spot signs of a skin rash, itching, blisters, swelling, or pain.

Pass the pepper. Capsaicin, the ingredient that makes red peppers hot, also numbs pain and soothes inflammation. The effect is only temporary, so you have to keep using the cream to feel the benefits.

Just as peppers burn your tongue, capsaicin may burn your skin. If it becomes painful, wash off the cream with warm, soapy water.

Only use topical creams on your skin. Keep them away from your eyes, nose, mouth, and open wounds. Don't place bandages or heat on the creams, and stop using them if they irritate your skin.

Don't get burned on fake cures

With all the supplements for sale these days, it's hard to tell fact from fiction. Before you rush to the health store, get the facts on these popular arthritis remedies.

Glucosamine and chondroitin. Both compounds are made naturally in your body, helping it grow and strengthen cartilage. Some experts think getting more of them from supplements could slow or even repair the damage of mild to moderate osteoarthritis (OA).

A number of studies show glucosamine and chondroitin improve arthritis symptoms, but critics argue that the research has been poorly done and that some studies were actually funded by companies that make the supplements.

Talk with your doctor to see if these supplements are right for you. People in most studies took 1,500 milligrams (mg) of glucosamine each day — usually 500 mg three times a day, and 1,200 mg of chondroitin every day — or 400 mg three times a day. They work slowly, so you may have to take them for two or three months before you feel results.

Since glucosamine is made from crab shells, you may want to skip it if you're allergic to shellfish. It may also raise your blood sugar if you have diabetes, so monitor yourself carefully. Chondroitin, on the other hand, may upset your stomach and could thin your blood, so avoid using it alongside blood-thinning medications like warfarin or aspirin.

And buyers beware — some glucosamine and chondroitin supplements contain dangerous amounts of manganese. Humans only need about 2 mg of this trace mineral each day. More could be toxic. Play it safe and only take these supplements under a doctor's supervision.

SAM-e. S-adenosylmethionine, "sammy" to its fans, contains sulfur, a building block of the body's cells, including cartilage. In fact, healthy cartilage has two-thirds more sulfur than arthritic cartilage.

> **The B vitamins folate (B9) and cobalamin (B12) help your body use SAM-e. Fill your plate with folate-rich foods like fortified cereals and cobalamin-rich fish.**

As you age, your natural levels of SAM-e drop. Early studies show taking supplements may lessen joint pain and increase your range of motion as well as nonsteroidal anti-inflammatory drugs (NSAIDs) like ibuprofen or aspirin — without the side effects. Many health experts recommend getting 600 mg of

SAM-e each day for the first two weeks, then lowering the dose to 400 mg a day thereafter.

More research needs to be done, so talk with your doctor before taking this supplement. If you don't notice an improvement after the first month, see your doctor about changing your dosage or trying a different treatment.

> Are your joints frozen stiff come morning? Snuggle up in a sleeping bag to trap your body heat and help keep your joints warm all night.

MSM. Its full name is methylsulfonylmethane, but you can call it MSM. This sulfur-based compound is found in foods from tomatoes and corn to tea and coffee. As a supplement, it has been used to treat many conditions, from allergies to arthritis.

Researchers know little about how MSM fights OA. It seemed to relieve arthritis symptoms in eight out of 10 people in a recent study.

So far, it hasn't caused serious side effects, but you should discuss this supplement with your doctor before taking it. For the most benefit, experts recommend a whopping 2,000 to 3,000 mg of MSM a day for at least six weeks.

Guggul. This herb has long been used to treat arthritis, inflammation, and other illnesses in Ayurvedic medicine, the ancient medical practice of India.

In animal studies, it has soothed swollen joints as well as ibuprofen and hydrocortisone. In a study at Southern California University, a 67-year-old woman with knee OA took 500 mg of guggul three times a day. After three months, she had less knee pain and more flexible joints.

Treating OA with guggul is still experimental in the Western world, so see your doctor before trying it yourself.

Cat's claw. This Amazon herbal remedy seems to work as both an antioxidant and an anti-inflammatory, throwing OA a double punch. People in a recent study took either a placebo pill or 100 mg of freeze-dried cat's claw once a day. Within four weeks, those who received the herb felt less joint pain.

Some evidence suggests it could also protect your stomach from the side effects of NSAIDs.

The supplement used in this study was stronger than those sold in stores, so you might not experience the same results. Talk with your doctor if you're considering this herb to relieve your OA, and discuss the proper dosage.

Pop to stop arthritis

Crack away! Popping your joints may prevent osteoarthritis.

Most people believe cracking your knuckles – or any other joint – can cause arthritis. Dr. Tyler Cymet, Assistant Professor of Internal Medicine at Johns Hopkins University, is out to change people's minds. "A lot of the research is old, and a lot of what we teach people is contradictory."

"It's the use of the joint that's healthy," he explains. "The more you use it, the less likely you are to develop problems in the joint."

Far from damaging them, Cymet believes popping joints helps them move more smoothly and gives them a healthy workout.

On the other hand, joints that constantly crack are a hallmark of osteoarthritis. So when is a crack healthy and when does it signal disease? Healthy joints generally release a single, loud pop, says Cymet, while diseased ones tend to crunch.

See your doctor if you think you have osteoarthritis. He can test you and prescribe the best treatment.

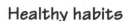

Healthy habits

You need a well-rounded game plan to win the war against osteoarthritis (OA). Try these tips to tackle this disease once and for all.

Shed extra pounds. Being overweight puts pressure on your joints. Lose those love handles, and you could improve your arthritis or even prevent it.

Get moving. Stronger muscles can mean stronger joints and less chance of OA, especially in your knees. Talk with your doctor about trying gentle exercises, like swimming and walking, and follow his advice.

Treat your tootsies right. Choose shoes with enough support to cushion your joints, and consider using wedge inserts. People in one study found that putting a 5-degree wedge in their shoes eased pressure on their knees without affecting their movement.

Seek out support. Learning about arthritis and sharing your worries with other people who have it can reduce pain and make for better living. Call the Arthritis Foundation at 1-800-283-7800 or visit their Web site at www.arthritis.org to find a group near you.

CHAPTER 28 *Osteoporosis*

What is osteoporosis? Osteoporosis is a disease where bones grow more weak and brittle over time.

Who develops it? Although osteoporosis mostly affects women, 20 percent of those with this condition are men. You have a higher risk of osteoporosis if you are Caucasian or Asian, have a family history of osteoporosis, experienced menopause before 45, are short and thin, are a current or recovering alcoholic, have no children, smoke, or have a low-calcium diet.

What are the symptoms? Occasionally, symptoms may include a stooped posture or lower back pain. But often people with osteoporosis have no symptoms until they suffer a fractured or broken hip, arm, or wrist, and are diagnosed with an X-ray or bone density test.

Look for calcium in all the right places

Say good-bye to the idea milk and other dairy products are the only sources of calcium. A new soft drink called MOOM is one of many options available to help you get more of this bone-building nutrient. Sure, you can still drink milk for calcium, but some folks can't eat dairy products, and some simply don't like them. That's where other choices – like MOOM – may help.

Developed at South Dakota State University, MOOM is a caffeine-free orange soft drink that gives you the same calcium and minerals as a glass of milk.

Although it takes its name from the fact that it's Made Out Of Milk (MOOM), this drink won't weigh you down with milk's fat and protein. Even better, some people who can't tolerate milk can drink MOOM with no trouble. So far MOOM isn't widely available, but its producers hope to change that.

Meanwhile, try to get more calcium – according to the Institute of Medicine, most American teenagers and adults aren't getting even the recommended daily amount. In fact, women of all age groups are, on average, 500 milligrams (mg) short. This is true even though calcium-fortified foods are now widely available. Adults under 50 only need 1,000 mg of calcium per day, but seniors need 1,200 mg.

Get lots of calcium regularly and you can:

- reduce bone loss.

- build stronger bones.

- lower your risk of fracture.

- delay – or even avoid – the crippling effects of osteoporosis.

Beware of second-class sources. Some foods contain a lot of calcium, but your body can't absorb and use it. Don't discard them from your diet. You can still gain other nutrients – just don't rely on them as your main source of this vital bone-builder.

- Many calcium-rich foods also contain a natural compound called oxalate. This traps most of the calcium and keeps your body from using it. So even if you eat loads of calcium-packed spinach, it contains enough oxalate that you won't benefit from the calcium. Other calcium misers include cranberries, rhubarb, and chard. Sweet potatoes and dried beans may leave you deprived of calcium as well.

- Another calcium bandit is a form of phosphorus called phytate. It lurks in fiber-rich foods like nuts, grains, raw beans, and some soy foods. Although phytates snare much less calcium than oxalates, they can still keep you from getting 100 percent of the calcium you expect.

Win with calcium champions. Remember calcium doesn't just mean dairy. Experts say, for instance, you can get just as much calcium from orange juice with added calcium citrate as from good old-fashioned milk. Here are other ways to get more calcium your body can use.

- Eat from a wide variety of calcium-filled foods including sardines and salmon with bones, shellfish, fortified commercial cereals, rice, stewed tomatoes, broccoli, and papayas.

- Need a calcium treat? Eat a little blackstrap molasses.

- For a portable, no-fuss snack with a calcium boost, try raisins, dates, or dried figs.

- If you decide to supplement, take two or three doses during the day, rather than one single dose. This way you won't get more calcium than your body can absorb at one sitting. According to research, a good calcium carbonate supplement can provide as much absorbed calcium as milk.

- To be able to use calcium, your body needs some vitamin D. What's more, high vitamin D levels are linked with all-round good bone health. For more on how this nutrient is linked to bone health, read on.

Boost your bone health with vitamin D

Your body can easily make vitamin D on its own if you get out in the sun regularly. In spite of that, vitamin D deficiency is more common – and more dangerous to your bone health – than you may realize.

Get the bottom line on better bones. Without vitamin D, your digestive tract is unable to absorb calcium from the foods you eat. When that happens, your body senses the calcium deficiency and triggers special cells to snatch some from your bones. While this helps your body get enough calcium for its other needs, it weakens your skeleton. The bottom line is, you need calcium and vitamin D together to build and strengthen your bones.

Know when you are at risk. Rickets – a bone condition caused by lack of vitamin D – was a major public health problem in the United States before 1930. Then, producers began fortifying milk with vitamin D and rickets disappeared – or so it seemed. Today, many experts believe diseases like rickets and osteoporosis are on the rise because there are still people at risk of vitamin D deficiency.

> Before you try vitamin D supplements or cod liver oil, check with your doctor. Too much vitamin D from these sources can be toxic.

"This deficiency typically occurs in elderly housebound individuals and in nursing home residents," explains Terrence Diamond, Associate Professor of Medicine at Australia's University of New South Wales. Yet according to Diamond who's done extensive research in vitamin D, if you are high-risk, you can become deficient even in sunny Australia.

In fact, Diamond's research team discovered severe vitamin D deficiency in over 60 percent of women at risk. They also found high bone turnover – a possible sign of bone loss – in 46 percent. Here's why some people are at risk.

- Many areas of the world receive less sunshine than others because of weather conditions or higher latitudes. In places like Canada, for instance, winters are long and days are short. For many months out of the year, people have fewer chances to get the sunlight their skin needs to make vitamin D. That's why Canadian researchers spent a year studying healthy residents of Calgary, a city in western Canada. At one or more times during the year, at least 34 percent had vitamin D levels bordering on deficiency.

- Diamond explains that if you avoid the sun or use sunscreen frequently, you are at risk. "The strong marketing campaign by the Cancer Council in Australia to apply blockout and avoid sunlight because of the high incidence of skin cancers, will almost certainly in the long-term result in a resurgence of vitamin D deficiency."

- Skin that has lots of pigment – or color – in it is less efficient at manufacturing vitamin D than lighter colored skin.

- Deficiency may sneak up on seniors in two ways. Your digestive system's ability to absorb vitamin D from food and your skin's ability to convert vitamin D both decline as you age.

- If you are lactose intolerant – can't digest milk products – you may come up short since you are less likely to get vitamin D from dairy foods.

- Vitamin D is a fat soluble vitamin. That means if you suffer from a condition that limits your ability to absorb fat – like liver disease, Crohn's disease, sprue, and others – you won't get enough D.

Learn how to mend a deficiency. If you need more vitamin D, here's what to do.

- Eat more cold-water fish like salmon, sardines, and herring.

- Eat more D-fortified foods such as ready-to-eat cereals, and milk and other dairy products.

- Eat a boiled egg occasionally. There's vitamin D in the yolk.

- Get just a little sun. Diamond recommends 20 to 30 minutes of sunlight three times a week on your face, hands, and legs.

Look to the future. University of Wisconsin scientists have discovered a new vitamin D compound called 2MD. In animal and lab tests, it seems to trigger the formation of new bone without side effects. Although 2MD has not been tested on humans, experts hope it could eventually reverse bone loss and increase bone density in people suffering from osteoporosis.

Stay strong with blue-ribbon nutrients

Like a giant broom, salt can sweep calcium out of your body. So even if you eat plenty of foods rich in calcium and vitamin D, you can sabotage your bones by eating too much salt. That's why you need the extra protection you can get from some of calcium's bone-building buddies.

Pick a peck of potassium. "For women at risk of osteoporosis, eating more fruits and vegetables is a simple way to help prevent the adverse effects of a typical American high-salt diet," says Deborah Sellmeyer, M.D., author of a study out of the University of California, San Francisco.

Experiment with salt substitutes including herbs, spices, and no-salt seasoning mixes.

Sellmeyer gave extra potassium to postmenopausal women on a high-salt diet and then measured how much calcium they lost compared to women taking a placebo, an inactive pill. Those on potassium were able to hold on to more calcium. She concluded that even if you eat more salt than you should, adding high-potassium foods to your diet can help save your bones.

You also need potassium to help your body absorb calcium. Researchers have found that seniors who get lots of potassium have higher bone mineral density – a measure of bone strength.

Aim for 3,500 milligrams (mg) of potassium a day by eating at least five servings of potassium-packed foods like these.

Food	Potassium
Potato, baked with skin, no salt	1081 mg
Halibut, 5 1/2 ounces, grilled	916 mg
Winter squash, 1 cup, baked, no salt	896 mg

Prunes, 1 cup, stewed, no sugar	828 mg
Papaya, 5 inches long	781 mg
Lima beans, 1/2 cup, boiled, no salt	478 mg
Banana, medium	467 mg

KO osteo with vitamin K. Research suggests you can reduce your risk of hip fracture if you get over 100 micrograms (mcg) of vitamin K each day. Not getting enough, on the other hand, has been linked to poor bone mineral density.

As a minimum, senior men should get 120 mcg of vitamin K and senior women need 90 mcg. Here are some foods that can give you this bone-supporting vitamin.

Food	Vitamin K
Kale, 1 cup, raw	410 mcg
Broccoli, 1/2 cup, cooked	210 mcg
Spinach, 1 cup, raw	120 mcg
Pistachios, 3 1/2 ounces	70 mcg
Kiwi, large, without skin	25 mcg
Canola oil, 1 tbsp	20 mcg

Vitamin K is associated with chlorophyll in foods, so pick the greenest veggies you can find for rich sources. Remember not to freeze these foods since this may destroy their vitamin K content. In addition, avoid extra vitamin K if you're on a blood thinner like Warfarin. This vitamin helps your blood clot and may counter this kind of drug.

Munch on more magnesium. According to the National Institute of Arthritis and Musculoskeletal and Skin Diseases, osteoporosis is responsible for more than 300,000 hip fractures every year. The good news is, the more magnesium you get, the stronger your hipbones.

If you're a man over 50, try for at least 420 mg of magnesium per day. Woman over 50 need a minimum of 320 mg. Grains, nuts, seeds, and legumes are all good sources but here are some other foods you might want to try.

Food	Magnesium
Halibut, 5 1/2 ounces, grilled	170 mg
Tropical trail mix, 1 cup	134 mg
Oat bran muffin, 2 ounces	89 mg
Spinach, 1/2 cup, boiled, no salt	79 mg
Black beans, 1/2 cup, cooked, no salt	60 mg

Favor your bones with phosphorus. Most of your body's supply of this mineral is in your bones where it binds with calcium to form a compound that makes them stronger. Many studies suggest that low phosphorus levels could mean both bone loss and calcium loss.

Ordinarily phosphorus is easy to absorb and is widely available in foods. Seniors, however, are less likely to get adequate phosphorus from their diet. In one study, 10 percent of women 60 to 80 years old got less than 70 percent of the recommended amount. On top of that, research out of Creighton University shows that some calcium supplements may limit your ability to absorb phosphorus.

If you are an older adult or if you take calcium supplements, it's a good idea to check with your doctor to determine whether you need more phosphorus.

Food	Phosphorus
Halibut, 5 1/2 ounces, grilled	453 mg
Salmon, 5 1/2 ounces, grilled	428 mg
Sunflower seeds, 1/4 cup, dry roasted with salt	370 mg
Lentils, 1 cup, boiled, no salt	356 mg
Cottage cheese, 1 cup, low-fat	341 mg
Ricotta cheese, 1/2 cup, part-skim	225 mg

Men need bone protection, too

In the United States alone, about 2 million men suffer from osteoporosis. Yet recent research shows they're not receiving treatment for the disease – even after suffering bone fractures.

In a study of over 300 seniors admitted to a Houston hospital with hip fractures due to osteoporosis, about 27 percent of the female patients were prescribed bone-building medication. Yet less than 5 percent of the male patients received similar treatment.

When doctors suspect osteoporosis, they use bone mineral density (BMD) scans to confirm the disease. Only 11 percent of the men studied had a BMD scan within five years of leaving the hospital – compared to 27 percent of women.

Until the medical community takes a more active role in diagnosing and treating male osteoporosis, you'll need to take on the responsibility of saving your bones yourself.

Stack the odds with helpful foods. Don't wait until you suffer a hip fracture to protect yourself from osteoporosis. Start today with a diet high in grains and produce.

Boston scientists examined bone strength and eating habits of more than 900 seniors. Of all the men in the study, the ones who ate the most fruit, vegetables, and cereal had the strongest bones – even compared to men who ate more dairy.

Can you squeeze in another fruit or vegetable each day? One study found that every extra serving of vegetables or fruit men added to their daily menu meant a 1 percent increase in hip bone density – and a 5 percent lower risk of hip fracture.

Nibble on those nutrients. So what do these foods have that may help build up your bones? The researchers noticed the group of men on a high fruit, veggie, and cereal diet also had the highest intake of many nutrients known to resist osteoporosis – specifically vitamin C, vitamin K, magnesium, and potassium.

Learn how to get more. Dr. Chris Rosenbloom, registered dietician and Georgia State University professor, suggests ways to get that extra serving or two of fruits and vegetables into your day.

She says you don't always have to use fresh fruits. Canned, frozen, or dried are quick and easy ingredients for many dishes. "A bag of frozen blueberries is a great addition to hot cereal or frozen yogurt," she says. "Dried fruit mixes are easy to store and make a good afternoon snack."

Rosenbloom also offers some different ideas for incorporating fruit into meals or as a sweet, but healthy dessert. "Top frozen waffles with fruit or make dried fruit compotes as a topping for grilled chicken or fish. Bake an apple for dessert or learn to poach a pear."

"For vegetables," she says, "I suggest the 'sneak' method. Toss veggies into the boiling water when cooking pasta. Top a grilled chicken breast with a mild tomato-based salsa or grate vegetables like carrots, bell peppers, and onions into

gelatin-based salads. Bake a sweet potato and top it with cinnamon or make a vegetable plate for dinner on occasion
instead of a meat-based entree."

All these strategies are great for anyone who doesn't want to
spend time in the kitchen but still wants to boost bone strength.

From heart to bones – tea is tip-top

People who suffer a stroke have a higher risk of bone loss and
fractures, according to recent research. If you want to protect
yourself against both stroke and osteoporosis in one easy step,
try drinking the world's second most popular beverage – tea.

Take time for tea. Drinking tea over the long-term may be more
important to your bone health than how much you drink each
day. In fact, if you've been sipping regularly for more than 10
years, your spine, hip, and overall bone strength is probably
greater than it would be otherwise.

Although your body constantly casts off old bone cells and
replaces them with fresh new ones, this doesn't happen over-
night. Building good solid bone takes time.

Researchers from the National Cheng Kung University Hospital in Taiwan examined tea drinking habits and total body,
spine, and hip bone strength of over one thousand Chinese
men and women.

They found that people who drank tea at least once a week for
more than six years had better bone strength in the spine than
people who drank tea less often. What's more, people who
drank tea at least once a week for more than 10 years showed
better bone strength in the spine, hip, and total body than less
frequent tea drinkers.

Brew black, get green, or opt for oolong. Even though most tea
drinkers in the Chinese study preferred green or oolong tea,

those who drink black tea don't lose out. The researchers found no significant difference in bone mineral density between the three types of tea drinkers.

All types of tea provide fluoride, which can slow the progress of osteoporosis. In addition, certain flavonoids – natural plant chemicals – in tea have been proven to increase bone density. Tea's third benefit comes from its extracts which help keep calcium from leaching out of your bones.

Build more than just bone. Although the benefits of drinking tea may not show up in your bones right away, consider what else tea may do for you right now.

- Research suggests that an amino acid in tea may make your blood less sticky – lowering your chance of plaque buildup that can lead to heart disease and stroke.

- A study of almost 5,000 seniors showed a relationship between drinking tea and a reduced risk of heart attack.

- Natural chemicals in tea act as antioxidants – they hunt down and destroy molecules in your body that cause disease and cancer. In fact, green tea in particular is known to fight cancers of the breast, stomach, colon, and prostate.

- Both black and green tea may help you fend off skin damage from sunlight. With less skin damage, you may also resist wrinkles and reduce your chance of skin cancer.

Start drinking tea for your bones now and you may be able to look forward to a longer, healthier life.

Bones of contention: the protein and soy debate

Just what would you do to prevent bone loss after menopause? After all by age 65 many women have lost half their skeletal mass. Would you try a controversial remedy? If you're on hormone replacement therapy (HRT) you may be walking a thin line between healing and harming. But what about a more natural solution – say foods or natural supplements?

Be prudent with protein. Protein is about as basic to human life and as natural a food source as you'll find. Yet neither the amount of protein a mature woman needs for good bone health nor the most beneficial source – animal or vegetable – is so cut and dried.

There are two schools of thought – protein strengthens your bones and protein weakens your bones.

Tufts University scientists say seniors who eat more protein while taking a calcium and vitamin D supplement can improve bone strength – even reverse bone loss. Although the generally recommended protein intake is 40 to 60 grams a day, those in the study averaged close to 80 grams per day. That's equal to a 5-ounce serving of poultry plus about a cup and a half of low-fat cottage cheese. They also took 500 milligrams of calcium citrate and 17.5 micrograms of vitamin D.

According to experts, it took a combination of these to bring on positive effects. "Our results suggest that a higher calcium intake is going to be protective against any adverse effects of protein on bone, and may allow protein to have a positive effect," says Bess Dawson-Hughes, M.D., lead author of the study and senior scientist at the Calcium and Bone Metabolism Laboratory at Tufts University.

In other words, when there is enough calcium in your diet, protein, whether from plant or animal sources, may help your body absorb the calcium better.

The anti-protein camp says for every extra gram of protein you eat, you lose up to 1.5 milligrams of calcium through your urine. In addition, one study found that older women who ate the most animal protein more than tripled their hip fracture risk.

Until this controversy is settled, eat a calcium-rich, well-rounded diet with protein from a variety of animal and vegetable sources. Include fish, lean meats, grains, low-fat dairy foods, nuts, eggs, and beans.

Set limits on soy. Do you tofu? Perhaps you used to but are now torn between the proven benefits of soy — reduced symptoms of menopause and lower risk of heart disease — and the suggested dangers — brain aging, senility, slowed thyroid function, and an increased risk of breast cancer.

Add to the controversy the impact a natural plant chemical in soy has on your bone health. Isoflavones seem to have a positive, negative, and even indifferent effect on bone mineral density, depending on which scientific study you choose to believe.

Research out of University of North Carolina's School of Public Health and Medicine shows that young women who took an isoflavone-loaded soy supplement did not change bone strength.

Perhaps, say the experts, these young women have too much estrogen to benefit from soy's isoflavones. After all, bone loss in older women may be linked to plummeting estrogen levels that accompany menopause.

Yet there are studies of older women which show soy isoflavones lowering bone loss and increasing bone strength.

The International Food Information Council Foundation, an independent food safety, nutrition, and health organization says it's not possible at this time to draw a clear conclusion regarding the effects and safety of soy on long-term bone health. Until more information is available, play it safe — limit soy.

Healthy habits

Protect your bones with these lifestyle strategies.

- Exercise with weights three times per week and you could increase the density – or strength – of your hip bone, a typical area of fractures and major disability in seniors. Called high-intensity resistance exercise, this type of program includes leg presses, overhead presses, and specific back exercises. Talk to your doctor before beginning this type of exercise.

- Help all your bones with regular, everyday exercise like yard work, stair-climbing, hiking, jogging, walking, gardening, or dancing.

- Improve your balance and avoid falls by trying a tai chi exercise class.

- Ask your doctor about any medication – or health condition – that could cause or increase bone loss. If you are at risk, check your bone mineral density (BMD).

- The National Osteoporosis Foundation recommends BMD screening for women over 65, women past menopause who have had a bone fracture, and women who have taken hormone replacement therapy for a long time.

- Stop smoking and drink alcohol only in moderation.

Prostate cancer

What is prostate cancer? Prostate cancer occurs when cells in the prostate gland, where men's bodies make and store semen, divide and grow until they form a tumor.

Who gets it? The risk increases with age and is greater for men with a family history of the disease. Additional risk for black men and bald men may be related to higher levels of the male hormone androgen.

What are the symptoms?

- frequent, difficult, or painful urination
- dribbling
- blood in the urine
- painful ejaculation
- hip or back pain

Protect your prostate with a potent diet

If you are one of those men who typically gets most of his calories from fat, sugar, and beer, your prostate may be in grave danger. Unless you change your diet, you may put yourself at risk for prostate cancer.

"The bottom line," says Dr. Alan Kristal of the Fred Hutchinson Cancer Research Center in Seattle, "is that if you eat a lot of vegetables, you can cut your risk of prostate cancer by about 45 percent."

Here are a few of the most powerful cancer-fighting plant foods.

Cruciferous vegetables. In Kristal's study, men who ate as little as three half-cup servings of cruciferous vegetables — such as broccoli, cauliflower, and cabbage – per week reduced their risk of prostate cancer by 41 percent compared to men who ate fewer than one serving per week.

> The form of vitamin E that best protects the prostate — gamma-tocopherol — isn't the kind people usually buy in pills. Get the protective kind from natural sources like almonds, eggs, and olive oil.

Tomato sauces. Ketchup, spaghetti sauce, and other cooked tomato sauces contain high amounts of lycopene. Men with the most of this phytochemical in their bloodstream, according to a Yale University study, were 35 percent less likely to get prostate cancer than those with the least.

This amazing nutrient may protect you from five other cancers, colon, stomach, lung, esophagus, and throat, as well.

You can get smaller amounts of lycopene from fresh tomatoes, watermelon, and pink grapefruit. But keep an eye out for red autumn olive berries, which recent tests show have 17 percent more lycopene than tomatoes. Although they are mainly fed to birds, people can eat them, too.

Citrus fruits. Pectin, another helper in your fight against prostate cancer, is abundant in oranges, lemons, grapefruit, and tangerines. It's best to eat the whole fruit, not just the juice, because most of the pectin is in the meat and membranes.

Apples, red onions, tea, and grapes. What these foods have in common is quercetin, a flavonoid that protects against prostate cancer. You can also get it from beans, dark green vegetables, and citrus fruits.

Herbs and spices. Include parsley – fresh or dried – in salads and other dishes. This simple herb slashes your risk of both breast and prostate cancer. Also, remember to stir prostate-friendly garlic into soups and sauces.

Add some curry dishes to your diet, too. The spice turmeric, which gives curry its yellow color, contains an ingredient called curcumin, which may be another cancer fighter.

Nuts, seeds, and grains. Eat almonds and walnuts for vitamin E, whole grains for both vitamin E and selenium, and pumpkin seeds for zinc. All these nutrients are key to prostate health.

If you are thinking it might be simpler to get all these potent prostrate protectors in a pill, think again.

"Vegetables – all food, actually – contain many biologically active components," Kristal points out. These components work together in complex ways, so it's important to eat a wide variety of vegetables.

"I don't think pills will take the place of eating a good diet," he says, "at least not in my lifetime."

Is this test necessary?

Autopsies show many men die of something else without knowing they have prostate cancer. Treatment can be risky, so some health experts recommend delaying testing unless there are symptoms. Others say a man has a right to know and then can decide whether to get treatment or practice "watchful waiting."

Limit fat, calcium to keep cancer in check

Fatty steaks, chops, and burgers, downed with glasses of whole milk, may seem like a manly diet. But "real men" don't want problems with their prostate. Fortunately, a few changes to your diet can make a big difference, especially if you are in the early stages of prostate cancer.

"Our findings clearly show decreased risk for late-stage disease in men with diets that are low in fat and moderate in calcium," says Dr. Alan Kristal, "perhaps because these diets slow progression of prostate cancer into more aggressive disease."

The changes he suggests, based on research at the Fred Hutchinson Cancer Research Center in Seattle, may also reduce the risk of cancer coming back again after treatment.

> Some men find that saw palmetto and stinging nettle help reduce an enlarged prostate. For others, African plum tree reduces inflammation and increases bladder output. Talk to your doctor about these herbs.

Reduce total calories. The Hutchinson study found men who ate the fewest calories each day reduced by half their risk of getting prostate cancer – and of it reaching an advanced stage – when compared to men who ate the most calories.

Eat less fat. While some think fat intake isn't such an important health issue, Kristal disagrees. He and his fellow researchers found that men who ate lower-fat diets – no more than 30 percent of their daily calories coming from fat – cut their risk of late-stage cancer in half.

Both saturated fat, the kind you get in meats and dairy foods, and monounsaturated fats (MUFAS), from olive and peanut oils, were equally associated with advanced cancer risk in this study. Certain polyunsaturated oils, like canola and safflower, were not.

In another study, however, men who ate one teaspoon of olive, canola, or peanut oil a day had a 50 percent lower risk of prostate cancer than the men who didn't use these MUFAs at all. Of course, all fats are high in calories, so go easy, even on the healthiest ones.

Unlike other research, Kristal's study didn't find the omega-3 fatty acids of fish like salmon and tuna to be protective against prostate cancer. But another study finds flaxseed, the richest plant source of omega-3 fatty acids, promising.

Cut back on calcium. Your body needs some calcium, but too much can double your risk of advanced prostate cancer. The Hutchinson study found this true of men with the highest intake – more than 1,200 milligrams (mg) per day, the equivalent of four or more glasses of milk – when compared to those who got less than half that amount.

> Studies suggest that soy isoflavones make radiation treatment for prostate cancer more effective. Tests are currently under way to see if eating soy foods before treatment helps.

It may be that calcium interferes with your body's use of vitamin D, which seems to protect against prostate cancer. Results were the same whatever the source – dairy foods, fortified juices, or supplements.

Healthy habits

Keep your prostate healthy with a few simple lifestyle changes to go along with your healthy diet.

- Get regular exercise.
- Maintain a healthy weight.
- Relax to reduce stress.
- Spend time in sunlight for vitamin D.
- Take NSAIDS – with your doctor's approval.

CHAPTER 30 *Rheumatoid arthritis*

What is rheumatoid arthritis? Rheumatoid arthritis (RA) is an autoimmune disease where your immune system attacks your joints, damaging your cartilage, bones, and even affecting organs like your heart and lungs.

Who gets it? Only about 1 to 2 percent of people develop RA, but women are three times as likely to get it as men. It tends to run in families and most often strikes people between the ages of 20 and 40.

What are the symptoms?

- stiff, swollen, warm, and painful joints
- fatigue, weakness, and weight loss
- low-grade fever
- joints that become knobby and hard to move

Oil up to ease achy joints

Putting oil in a car keeps the engine running smoothly, so why wouldn't it do the same for your body? Natural oils in everyday foods can keep your joints moving smoothly when rheumatoid arthritis (RA) starts to slow you down.

Look at olives in a new way. The golden oil squeezed from them could ward off rheumatoid arthritis. Olive oil is loaded with healthful monounsaturated fatty acids that relieve inflammation while its antioxidants nab free radicals before they can harm your body. In fact, olive oil beat out all other foods in banishing RA during a study in Greece. Out of over 300 people, those who ate the least olive oil more than doubled their risk for RA compared with people who got three or more tablespoons a day.

Not all olive oils are created equal. Look for the kind labeled "extra virgin." It comes from the first press of the olives and has the most health benefits.

Make your own anti-arthritis meal by slicing and stir-frying fresh vegetables in olive oil, or using it as a base for salad dressings. Reach for it instead of butter, margarine, or other vegetable oils when you cook. Use a little every day, and you could soon feel the difference.

Feast on flax. Oil from this plant is a proven friend to arthritis sufferers. It helps control cytokines, compounds in your body that cause inflammation, and next to fish it's the best source of joint-soothing omega-3 fatty acids.

Experts suggest you get one tablespoon a day for every 100 pounds you weigh. Start with a smaller amount if you have food allergies, and slowly add it to your diet. Try pouring it on salads and vegetables for a flavorful treat, but don't use it to fry foods. It breaks down in very high heat and could become more harmful than healthy.

Look for flaxseed oil in health food stores and supermarkets, and always check the expiration date for freshness. You can store it in your refrigerator for up to two months, or in your freezer for up to a year. Just remember to throw it out if it starts to smell too fishy.

Pamper yourself with pumpkin seeds. Pumpkins aren't just fall ornaments. The "green gold" made from their seeds is a tasty oil with a store of omega-3, selenium, vitamin E, beta carotene, and other antioxidants sure to get your sore joints moving.

Finding this oil can be tricky. Originally from Austria, it's slowly appearing on shelves in other countries. Health and gourmet food stores are your best bets, but your local supermarket may surprise you by carrying it, too. You can cook with pumpkin seed oil, or pour it raw on salads for a unique, nutty flavor.

Remember no matter how healthy they are, oils are high in calories. Use them in moderation to add a dash of flavor, knowing that with every mouthful, you're taking a bite out of RA.

Remarkable way to relieve joint pain

Painful joints? You may find real pain relief naturally just by balancing two nutrients in your diet – one that helps calm inflammation and another that can aggravate it.

Omega-3 and omega-6 are two fatty acids your body needs to run smoothly, but here's the important catch – you need them in the right proportions.

Omega-6 is easy to find in modern diets. It's plentiful in vegetable oils, eggs, meat, milk, and fried or processed foods. Omega-3, on the other hand, is a rarer bird, showing up in olive and canola oils, fatty fish, nuts, seeds, and wheat germ – foods most people don't eat often enough.

> **Pills made from uncooked chicken collagen are all the rage, but do they work? "We're studying it, but the results aren't in," says Harvard researcher David Trentham.**

As a result, you could be getting up to 25 times more omega-6 than omega-3. Eating a diet like this is just asking for pain. That's because too much omega-6 in your body feeds inflammation, whereas omega-3 helps relieve it.

Balancing these two nutrients may feel like walking a tight rope, but the results could be worth it. A better ratio of fatty acids may keep your immune system healthy, ward off diseases like RA, and reduce already-active inflammation.

Reining in these ratios is simple. First, try replacing vegetable oils like corn, safflower, soybean, and cottonseed with olive or canola oils when you cook. Next, cut back on processed and fast foods, and look for ways to fit in more cold-water fish such as albacore tuna, salmon, mackerel, herring, bluefish, or striped bass. Ideally, you'll lower that ratio to about two to four times more omega-6 than omega-3.

Try these other time-tested nutrition tips to break the grip of rheumatoid arthritis.

Stock up on selenium. This mineral is also an anti-inflammatory, and it just may protect you from developing RA. Out of 18,000 people in Finland, those with the lowest levels of this nutrient were most at risk for a type of RA called rheumatoid factor-negative arthritis.

Getting your share of selenium is as easy as strolling through the supermarket. Just shop for a variety of seafood and poultry, as well as mushrooms, whole grains, and raw fruits and vegetables. Be careful about supplements. People over the age of 51 only need 55 micrograms (mcg) of selenium a day. More than that could be toxic.

Two tablespoons of shelled sunflower seeds provide almost half the E you need in a day.

Defeat disease with vitamin E. This natural antioxidant could play a role in preventing RA. In the same Finnish study, people who developed rheumatoid arthritis tended to have low levels of vitamin E.

Many cooking oils are rich in vitamin E, but be sure to pick oils like olive and canola that have more omega-3 fatty acids than omega-6. You can also find vitamin E in dark leafy greens, fortified cereals, wheat germ, nuts, and seeds. Think twice before taking supplements. Some experts believe too much vitamin E may actually worsen autoimmune diseases like RA.

Add on other antioxidants. Dangerous compounds called free radicals can run rampant in RA sufferers, leading experts to believe these trouble-makers contribute to joint damage. To fight back, you need the protective powers of antioxidants.

Many nutrients, like selenium and vitamin E, act as antioxidants in your body. Resveratrol, a flavonoid mainly found in red grapes and red wine, is another. Making a meal out of fresh fruits and vegetables will give you a variety of antioxidants and help you turn the tables on RA.

Honesty is the best policy

Humbleness and modesty may be heavenly traits, but it pays to be honest about your health.

Women are three times more likely than men to develop rheumatoid arthritis (RA), but they tend to downplay their symptoms to their doctors.

This is a dangerous game of deception because the disease does most of its damage early on. The longer it goes untreated, the worse the damage to your joints.

It's important to be open with your doctor so you can fight RA together. Let him know how bad the pain, tiredness, and other symptoms are, and how often you have them. You'll help him prescribe the right treatment, and he'll help you move toward a life without RA.

What you drink can affect your joints

Drink to your health, but choose wisely. Some beverages may protect you from rheumatoid arthritis (RA), while others could put you at risk.

For more than 10 years, Dr. Ted Mikuls, an Assistant Professor at the University of Nebraska Medical Center, studied 30,000 women between the ages of 55 and 69, keeping track of all the beverages they drank. The results revealed surprising new twists in the RA plot and could affect you.

Duck the dangers of decaf. Women who drank four or more cups of decaffeinated coffee a day, in this study, were more than twice as likely to develop rheumatoid arthritis. Regular coffee, on the other hand, had no effect.

What's so dangerous about decaf? Strong chemicals were used to decaffeinate coffee up until the mid-1970s. The women may have unknowingly been consuming these chemicals for years.

Decaf today is mostly made using safer, water-based methods, so you don't necessarily need to cut back. "I wouldn't make that recommendation based on our single study," agrees Mikuls. So stay tuned and wait until experts know more about how it influences RA.

Tip your hat to tea. If you want to play it safe, ditch the coffee and switch to tea. Out of all the women in this study, those who drank at least three cups of tea a day were least likely to develop RA.

The secret could lie in tea's team of protective antioxidants and soothing anti-inflammatory agents, says Mikuls. His study didn't look at specific kinds of tea, but he says other studies have shown that "some teas, particularly the purified green teas" may dampen inflammation. So pour yourself a cup of tea, and say cheers to your health.

Make way for milk. The vitamin D in fortified milk could make a difference if you have RA. Animal studies show it may quiet inflammation, and it's crucial in protecting your bones from osteoporosis, an ailment common in people with rheumatoid arthritis.

But can this vitamin prevent RA in the first place? Mikuls believes it might. In the study, researchers found that high levels of vitamin D offered some protection from developing this painful disease.

Some experts warn milk may aggravate arthritis in people with certain food allergies. If you're worried, turn to other sources for your daily dose of vitamin D, like a few minutes of sunshine or fresh seafood such as shrimp and salmon.

Keep in mind vitamin D can be toxic in large amounts, so check with your doctor before taking supplements.

Uncover allergies to control arthritis

Food allergies could be aggravating your arthritis. The sneaky suspects – gluten and lectin, two plant proteins found in grains like wheat, oats, barley, and rye.

Lectin may prompt your immune system to attack your joints, the problem in rheumatoid arthritis (RA).

Scientists aren't sure how gluten contributes, but past studies show eating a strict gluten-free diet may help some people with RA.

You'll find lectin mostly in grains, cereals, and legumes. Gluten hides in many grains as well as the foods made with them – flour, bread, sauces, gravies, candies, and even some alcoholic drinks.

You'd have to give up a lot to avoid them, but feeling better could be worth the sacrifice.

Special diets don't work for everyone. Some experts warn the more severe your arthritis or the longer you've had it, the less likely changing your diet will help.

Still, it could be worth a try. Talk with your doctor about whether food allergies could play a role in your arthritis.

Eat to defeat related diseases

Living with rheumatoid arthritis (RA) means you need to protect yourself against other illnesses that tag along with this disease. The sooner you start, the healthier you'll be.

Heart disease. It's the main cause of death among people with RA. Having arthritis can limit your physical activity and lead to weight gain, while inflammation can accelerate plaque buildup in your blood vessels.

Add in the high cholesterol and triglyceride levels and low HDL cholesterol that tend to go with RA, and you see how this arthritis sets the stage for heart disease.

> **Talk with your doctor about taking small, daily doses of aspirin in addition to other RA drugs to offset your risk for heart disease.**

Luckily, you can take steps now to control your weight, lower your cholesterol, and lengthen your life. First, cut back on saturated fats by choosing low-fat dairy products and lean cuts of meat. Then, fit in more unsaturated fats from foods like olive oil, nuts, or avocados. Last, get a little mild exercise several times a week.

Osteoporosis. Rheumatoid arthritis can hit your bones hard, doubling a woman's risk for osteoporosis. A Norwegian study found that taking steroids, having the rheumatoid factor, or being badly disabled by RA increased women's chances of developing osteoporosis.

Put the brakes on this bone disease with good nutrition. Aim to get 1,200 milligrams (mg) of calcium each day from foods like sardines, black-eyed peas, and low-fat milk, yogurt, and cheese.

Combine that with 10 micrograms (mcg) of vitamin D a day if you are between the ages of 51 and 70, or 15 mcg if you are over 70 years old. You can find vitamin D in salmon, shrimp, fortified milk, and a few minutes of sunshine on your skin. This vitamin can be toxic in high doses, so talk with your doctor before taking a supplement.

Gum disease. A positive attitude is important. But you better take care of your teeth, or you could lose that sunny smile. Gum disease is all too common among RA sufferers.

Inflammation and a confused immune system may affect your gums, or stiff arthritic joints could prevent people from brushing and flossing thoroughly.

Whatever the cause, try eating a well-balanced diet with plenty of calcium and vitamin C to strengthen your teeth, gums, and immune system. You'll find vitamin C in fruits and vegetables like oranges, strawberries, and broccoli, and calcium in dairy foods, small bony fish, and legumes.

Sjorgren's syndrome. Sjorgren's is an autoimmune disorder that sometimes accompanies rheumatoid arthritis. It causes your immune system to attack the glands that keep your mouth and eyes moist, resulting in a dry mouth, itching, burning eyes, and blurry vision.

You can moisten your mouth by sipping milk and chewing gum with a sugar substitute like Xylitol. See your doctor if you think you might have Sjorgren's syndrome. He can diagnose and treat it properly.

Celiac disease. This disorder can also appear alongside rheumatoid arthritis. It damages your small intestine, making it hard for your body to absorb nutrients from food. To promote healing, you'll have to rid your diet of gluten, a mixture of proteins found mostly in grains.

Tell your doctor if you develop symptoms of Celiac disease, such as weakness, weight loss, stomach bloating, bone pain, or diarrhea.

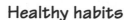

Healthy habits

Pain is no laughing matter, but it doesn't have to rule your life. Learn to manage your rheumatoid arthritis with this proven advice.

- Do everything you can to relieve your pain. Apply heat or cold to your joints, rest them, and take your medications the way your doctor prescribed.

- Go easy on yourself when your arthritis is acting up. Prioritize your activities. Do only the ones you must.

- Exercise when you can, but listen to your body. If your pain gets worse an hour after working out, you may not be ready for lots of physical activity.

- Rest up during flare ups. Aim to sleep at least 10 hours a day whether at night or with naps.

- Try to shift positions and stretch often while resting your joints. Leaving them bent for too long can damage the tissue around them and limit your movement even more.

CHAPTER 31 *Sinusitis*

What is sinusitis? Sinusitis is inflammation of the air pockets around your nose and eyes. When a cold or flu clogs your nose, it blocks the drainage of sinus fluids. The trapped mucus forms a perfect environment for bacteria or fungi to breed and cause infection.

Who gets it? About 37 million Americans get sinusitis every year. Those with colds or allergies are more at risk.

What are the symptoms?

- pressure around the bridge of your nose or eye sockets, especially in the morning or when leaning over
- low-grade fever with headaches or swollen eyes
- green, gray, or yellow mucus and postnasal drip
- ear or dental pain

Is it really sinusitis?

Figuring out what's causing your runny nose can be confusing. Colds, flu, allergies, and sinusitis all have similar symptoms. Stuffy nose, sneezing, coughing, sore throat, facial pressure, and fatigue occur in all four.

Only a doctor can say for sure which condition you have, but here are some clues to help you solve the mystery.

Cold or flu. Has someone in your family just been sick? Being around someone with a cold or flu increases your chances of getting it, too. Along with a stuffy nose and sneezing, you may have a fever and feel achy. Your nasal discharge should be clear or only slightly yellow. Colds generally last from three days to a week, while flu should clear up after 10 days or so.

Allergies. If your symptoms come around every year during allergy season or when you're exposed to dust or pets, it's pretty safe to assume you have allergies. What sets allergies apart is the itchiness in your eyes and nose.

Sinusitis. You should suspect you have sinusitis when your cold symptoms get worse and last longer than a week. Sinusitis may give you a headache first thing in the morning, painful sinus pressure at night, or pain when you bend over. Your nasal discharge might be yellowish green or gray and you may have a sore throat from postnasal drip.

There are two main kinds of sinusitis. Acute sinusitis usually follows a cold or flu and lasts less than a month. Chronic sinusitis can be caused by allergies or abnormalities in your nose. It's milder than the acute form, but it can last for several months.

If your fever climbs above 106 degrees Fahrenheit – or if your eyes get red and swollen, bulge out, or seem paralyzed – contact your doctor immediately. Sinusitis is rarely life threatening, but these symptoms could mean the infection is traveling to other parts of your body.

5 spicy solutions to sinus problems

Having an attack of sinusitis can be even more miserable than dealing with heart disease. A study showed that people with chronic sinus problems had more pain and less pleasure in their daily lives than those with back pain, heart disease, and other chronic conditions.

But you don't have to give in without a fight. Next time bacteria set up shop in your vulnerable sinuses, try these feisty foods to flush out your pipes in a hurry.

Give garlic a go. The smell of this bulb will keep more than just your friends away. The stinky compound in garlic, allicin, kills fungi and bacteria and gives your immune system a much needed boost. Experts recommend mincing one-half to three cloves a day to take advantage of garlic's antiseptic qualities. Garlic is best eaten fresh or just briefly heated – cook it too long and it loses its potency.

Slice open an onion. Garlic's relative, the common onion, can also fend off infection. You can relieve the congestion in your nose with this vegetable without even eating it. Just cut an onion in half and inhale deeply. You'll cry for joy as your sinuses clear.

Chop up some ginger. Like garlic, this aromatic rhizome may help nip a bacterial infection in the bud. At the very least, it will clear out mucus in your nose and soothe a sore throat. Steep three or four slices of fresh ginger root in a pint of hot water for a healing tea or eat a few cubes of the candied variety.

Sample some horseradish. If you've ever watched someone's face flush after eating this potent root, you can imagine how quickly it clears your sinuses.

Make sure you have some tissues handy when you brew a tea with a little grated horseradish and some honey. A little goes a long way, so keep your portions small. Too much of it may cause stomach upset and diarrhea.

Cook with cayenne. Cayenne is famous for cutting through sinus blockage. Spice up your meals with this numbing fire, but don't eat this pepper raw unless you're used to it. Wash your hands carefully after cutting it up. If you get it in your eyes, it will burn intensely.

Along with these hot and spicy cures, eat plenty of fruits and vegetables and drink lots of water to keep your sinuses moist. With your body prepared to fight off any sinus attack, you won't need to worry about sinusitis again.

Healthy habits

Keeping your sinuses moist and clear can disarm your sinusitis. Try these tips for sinus success.

- Dissolve half a teaspoon of salt in 8 ounces of warm water. Use a bulb syringe to gently flush your nose twice a day.

- Drape a warm, wet washcloth over your sinuses or lean over a steaming sink to clear up your airways.

- Don't blow your nose. This can send bacteria into your sinuses. Take an antihistamine instead.

- Let the tears come. Crying relieves stress and pent-up pressure in your sinuses.

- Hum a favorite tune. Swedish researchers found that humming can keep your sinuses clear and healthy.

- Exercise moderately to improve your air flow.

- Sleep with your head elevated to help your sinuses drain.

- Avoid smoke and other irritants such as wheat, wine, milk, and self-copying, or carbonless, paper.

- Don't use a nasal spray for more than three days in a row. It can cause even worse "rebound" congestion.

CHAPTER 32

Skin cancer

What is skin cancer? Skin cancer, the most common form of cancer, is an abnormal growth of cells on the skin. These tumors, if left untreated, may spread. The three main types of skin cancer are basal cell carcinoma, squamous cell carcinoma, and melanoma.

Who gets it? People with fair complexions, too much sun exposure, family history of skin cancer, history of sunburns early in life, or exposure to hazardous chemicals are at greater risk.

What are the symptoms?

- any changes in the size, color, shape, or border of a mole or other skin growth
- any open or inflamed wound that won't heal

'Tea' it up to save your skin

Do you thirst for ways to keep your skin youthful and cancer-free? Then try tea to bag extra protection for your skin.

Studies show tea helps your skin armor itself against harm from the sun's rays. And when you fend off skin cell damage, you may push away wrinkles and skin cancer as well.

Choose green or black tea. All teas are not created equal. Herbal teas may be healthy, but your skin will love black and green teas. Both kinds come from the *Camellia sinensis* plant, but black tea is fermented before packaging, while green tea is not.

One study suggests black tea, which gets its power from cancer fighters called theaflavins, protects you better than green tea.

Yet many studies show green tea is no slouch in the protection department, either. That's because it's loaded with antioxidants called catechins. These mighty substances neutralize the free radicals that can lead to tissue damage and disease.

Turn up the heat. Believe it or not, how you take your tea might make a difference in how well it protects your skin. Research from sun-drenched Arizona discovered that people who drank their black tea hotter and stronger had lower odds of getting skin cancer. These artful risk dodgers brewed their tea for two to seven minutes.

> **Avoid Earl Grey tea. It contains bergamot oil, which boosts your skin's sensitivity to sunlight. This raises your risk of skin damage and skin cancer.**

Decide about decaf. Unlike many herbal teas, black and green tea have caffeine. Of course, you can buy decaffeinated versions, but are they better for your skin? One animal study showed that decaffeinated tea still fought skin cancer, but was slightly less effective than caffeinated tea. A later mouse study suggested decaffeinated tea might be of little or no help. Regardless of which tea you choose, try to drink about three cups per day.

Add citrus for 'a-peel.' You can drive a wedge between your skin and harmful sunlight. Just make sure that wedge is made of lemon. Research shows that a substance called d-limonene in lemon, grapefruit, and orange peels may ward off cancer.

University of Arizona researchers found that adding citrus peel to your diet reduces your risk of skin cancer. Sipping hot black tea with citrus peel lowers your risk even more than drinking tea by itself.

Mix in some milk. You might think that adding milk to your tea would weaken the protection you get. Yet when Australian researchers put this to the test, they found that black tea with 10 percent whole milk still had an anti-cancer effect on mice. They also noticed a "dose response" — which means the more black tea you swig, the better.

Know tea's limits. One study of mice suggests that drinking tea does not protect you from a common skin cancer called basal cell carcinoma. It's not yet clear whether humans would see the same results. In the meantime, experts agree that green and black teas still help you avoid squamous cell carcinoma, another common skin cancer.

> **Drink green tea or rub it on your skin before or after any PUVA treatment. This combination of the drug psoralen and ultraviolet light, often used to treat psoriasis, increases skin cancer risk. Tea helps counteract it.**

Rub it in. You might suspect that tea would be more effective if you just rubbed it right on your skin. Some researchers have had the same idea. In a recent study, scientists painted a green tea catechin on mice daily for several weeks. The catechin seemed to suppress sun-related skin tumors.

On top of that, a small study discovered that rubbing green tea extract on human skin kept it from getting sunburned as badly as unprotected skin.

Don't ditch your sunscreen, though. Green tea won't block ultraviolet radiation the way sunscreen can. Instead, green tea seems to prevent skin cell damage, making your skin more resistant to sunburn.

Not surprisingly, some scientists recommend adding green tea to skin care products for extra protection. Before you buy sunscreen or other skin care products, check the ingredients. If they include green tea, you just might boost your defense against skin damage, skin cancer — and maybe even wrinkles.

Whether you get your tea from a teapot or a tube of sunscreen, you can help your skin win against cancer.

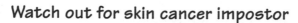

Watch out for skin cancer impostor

When you take off your favorite gold jewelry, you discover that the skin beneath has turned black. Is it skin cancer?

If the jewelry fits close to your skin and keeps it covered, the problem might just be black dermographism. This harmless condition happens when some ingredient in your jewelry rubs off on your skin.

Some say the chemicals in cosmetics, skin lotions, or even powder bring this on. Others suspect plain old sweat or natural chemicals put out by your skin might be the cause. Even the zinc oxide or titanium dioxide from sunscreen could be the guilty party.

Check with your doctor about the change in your skin – just to be sure it's not skin cancer. Meanwhile, don't use cosmetics or creams near this jewelry. If your problem really is black dermographism, that might be enough to make it go away.

Nurture modern skin with ancient food

Olive oil may be a famous food from ancient times, but it can safeguard your skin in the present day. Find out how this food can help.

Anoint your skin. Experts say your health may improve if you add olive oil to your diet. Now scientists from Japan suggest you might want to rub it on your skin, too.

Dr. Masamitsu Ichihashi, a dermatology professor at the Kobe University School of Medicine, worked with other researchers on a detailed study with mice. He found extra virgin olive oil may reduce the skin cell damage caused by sunlight. And less skin damage means you're more likely to resist skin cancer. The key is to use the right olive oil at the right time.

Wait until later. Apply olive oil after you come in from the sun, not before. Using olive oil as a sunscreen won't protect against the sun's ultraviolet-B (UVB) radiation. "Components of extra virgin olive oil may be destroyed by UVB radiation," Ichihashi says.

He explains that research has been done with one of olive oil's ingredients, oleuropein. When it was used as an after-sun lotion, oleuropein successfully limited sunlight's damage to skin cells. Yet, after oleuropein was exposed to UVB radiation, it no longer kept skin damage at bay. That indicates olive oil loses its ability to help you when it's drenched in sunlight.

So be sure to wear your favorite sunscreen, but don't add any soothing olive oil until your fun in the sun is done.

Insist on extra virgin. Remember to use extra virgin olive oil. Regular olive oil – and even virgin olive oil – won't do the job. Why? Apparently, they just don't have enough firepower.

> **Extra virgin olive oil comes from the first pressing of the olives. It has a lower acid content than either virgin or regular "pure" olive oil.**

"Super (extra) virgin olive oil seems to contain higher levels of antioxidants than simple virgin olive oil," Ichihashi says. That's important because antioxidants help shield your skin from the sun's damaging rays. In Ichihashi's study, mice treated with extra virgin olive oil fared better than those treated with virgin olive oil.

Spend the extra money for extra virgin olive oil. You might literally be saving your hide.

Include the food. Reach for the olive oil bottle again when you get hungry. Researchers from Australia's Monash University estimate that mixing two tablespoons of olive oil into your daily diet may help your skin. The monounsaturated fats in olive oil resist oxidation and protect your skin from sun damage.

"This study suggests that a lower fat diet may not be so good for your skin," says professor and lead researcher Mark Wahlqvist, "especially if the fat is derived primarily from animal foods high in saturated fat as opposed to antioxidant-rich plant foods such as olives, seeds, nuts, grains, legumes."

What's more, olive oil helps your skin add to its antioxidant stockpile. Your body needs fat in order to absorb certain antioxidants. So when you eat vegetables with olive oil, your body gets more antioxidant bang for its buck.

Olive oil can be an important part of your diet, as well as a helpful after-sun lotion. However you use it, this ancient food will make your skin feel like new.

Fight wrinkles naturally

Have you been wishing for cheap, natural alternatives to all those expensive anti-wrinkle potions? Here are eight ways to avoid wrinkles and look years younger.

- Pull out that olive oil bottle once more before bedtime. Just a few dabs of olive oil will make crow's feet fly away.

- For an anti-wrinkle mask, mix 2 tablespoons of honey with 2 teaspoons of milk. Apply this luxuriant blend to your face and neck and let it pamper your skin for 10 minutes. Then just rinse and enjoy the results.

- These six natural ingredients – lemon juice, lime juice, yogurt, papaya, mayonnaise, and cucumber – might also help you avoid wrinkles. Mix and match to see what works best for you.

Smooth out wrinkles before they start

Can the foods you eat protect your skin from sun damage and wrinkles? Researchers from two continents say they can.

See red for better skin. Lycopene puts the red in tomatoes, but it may also fight disease and tissue damage. In a small German study, scientists tested whether lycopene can help your skin resist the wrinkle-boosting harm caused by sunlight's ultraviolet (UV) radiation.

Research volunteers ate a daily dish of tomato paste and olive oil for 10 weeks. They got 16 milligrams of lycopene per day from this mixture. Other volunteers were given olive oil, but no tomato paste or lycopene.

Lycopene-eating volunteers showed 40 percent less sunburn than the other volunteers after week 10. The lycopene may have helped the skin defend itself against UV damage – and maybe fend off future wrinkles and skin cancer, too.

> While tomatoes and tomato products are the best sources of lycopene, you can find it in pink grapefruit, watermelon, and guava as well.

Just remember – this protection takes time to kick in. Lycopene eaters didn't see any skin protection until week 10.

Round up wrinkle fighters. "New evidence has emerged," scientists from Australia's Monash University announced, "that certain foods may protect sun-exposed skin from UV damage and wrinkling."

Led by Dr. Mark Wahlqvist and Dr. Antigone Kouris-Blazos, the research team examined the diets and skin wrinkling of 453 older adults from Greece, Sweden, and Australia.

Their study results suggest which foods may be associated with more wrinkles and which ones are wrinkle fighters. Here are some foods that might keep you looking years younger than your age.

- All fruits, but especially prunes, cherries, apples, olives, pears, melons, grapes, jam, and dried fruit. The researchers recommend two or three pieces of fruit per day.

- Nearly all vegetables, but especially leafy greens, spinach, eggplant, asparagus, celery, onions, leeks, and garlic. Try for at least five servings of vegetables, totaling 15 to 17 ounces, each day. If you're not sure how much that is, notice the ounces listed on cans or packages of vegetables and check the scale when you weigh fresh vegetables in the store.

- Lima beans, nuts, and other legumes

- Whole grain cereals

- Tea and water

- Olive oil

- Eggs, skim milk, low-fat yogurt, and low-fat cheese

- Fish, especially fatty fish such as sardines. The researchers estimate that a 3.5-ounce serving of fish twice a week might be the right amount for your skin. Your serving should be slightly larger than a deck of cards.

Aim for antioxidants. Why would these foods prevent wrinkles better than other foods? The Monash University researchers point out that the anti-wrinkle foods are generally high in antioxidants. "Foods which contain antioxidants may theoretically protect skin from UV damage," Wahlqvist says.

When skin is exposed to ultraviolet light, that light can harm skin cells and DNA. Compounds that prevent this damage are called antioxidants. Eating more antioxidant-rich foods raises the amount of wrinkle-resisting antioxidants in the skin. Fruits and vegetables are famous for their rich hoard of antioxidants, but even eggs and fish have some of their own.

"The main message from this study is that it may be possible to prevent premature aging and UV skin damage, and possibly even skin cancer, by including protective foods in your diet, by improving the fat quality of your diet, and by increasing your intake of monounsaturated fat," Wahlqvist says.

> **Eating fruit may not be the only way to prevent wrinkles. Look for fruit as an ingredient in skin care products and skin cleansers.**

Know your enemies. Getting more early wrinkles is as easy as pie – eating pie, that is. Here are the foods that may be linked to wrinkling.

- Most full-fat dairy foods including milk, margarine, butter, and ice cream. Your skin does not scream for ice cream.

- Meat and potatoes, especially red meat and processed meat

- Saturated fat

- High-sugar foods including soft drinks, cakes, and pastries. Kouris-Blazos recommends that you limit these to two or fewer servings per day. A single serving is two cookies, five lollipops, or two scoops of ice cream.

Look for opportunities to replace these foods with the foods that are more likely to prevent wrinkles.

Now that you can use both your sunscreen and your dinner plate to protect your skin, you have more power than ever to keep your skin youthful, healthy, and cancer-free.

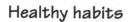

Healthy habits

You probably have no idea how much sunscreen to put on to protect your skin from the sun's harmful rays. Use the new "rule of nines" to help.

Grab your sunscreen and squeeze out a line from the tip of your index finger to the base. Make another sunscreen line on your middle finger, from tip to base. Researchers say this is just the right amount to cover 9 percent of your body. So, for each one of the following "9 percent" sections, use two fingers of sunscreen.

- head, neck, and face
- left arm
- right arm
- upper back
- lower back
- upper front (chest area)
- lower front (below the chest)
- left upper leg
- right upper leg
- left lower leg and foot
- right lower leg and foot

Remember to reapply sunscreen every two hours. When it comes to your skin, that's the best way to make sure you've got it covered.

CHAPTER 33 *Stroke*

What is a stroke? A stroke, or "brain attack," damages your brain the way a heart attack damages your heart. Some strokes are caused by blood clots that block the flow of blood to the brain (ischemic stroke), while others happen when a blood vessel in the brain ruptures (hemorrhagic stroke). As with a heart attack, fast action can save your life.

Who gets it? Two-thirds of all stroke victims are over 65 years old. Blacks are also at greater risk. Other risk factors include a personal or family history of stroke, high blood pressure, heart disease, and diabetes. Smoking and a lack of exercise are also major factors.

What are the symptoms? Numbness or weakness, especially on one side; confusion; trouble speaking or understanding; difficulty seeing; dizziness, loss of balance or coordination; and a sudden, severe headache.

8 remarkable ways to prevent a stroke

A stroke can strike suddenly, without warning. To protect yourself, make these fantastic foods part of your regular diet and stop stroke before it starts.

Go for garlic. No one herb or food can do it all, but this savory herb has earned the name "cure-all of the century." Scientists are just now discovering that this ancient remedy is effective against everything from stroke to ulcers — and has even been shown to help prevent breast cancer. Other herbs and foods shield your heart from a dangerous build-up of artery-clogging cholesterol. But garlic gives you the full anti-stroke package.

A substance in garlic called ajoene helps prevent blood from clumping and sticking together. That means it's less likely to clot. Garlic may also help lower your blood pressure and cholesterol, further reducing your risk for stroke. Pep up your next meal with this zesty life-saver.

Jazz it up with ginger. This spice comes with its own dynamic duo – gingerol and shogaol. These natural phytochemicals help prevent blood clots. Fresh or dried ginger will spice up your food and shore up your defenses against stroke.

Choose corn oil. A recent Japanese study found that linoleic acid, the kind found in corn oil, might lower your risk for ischemic stroke. Researchers suspect it works by lowering blood pressure and preventing platelets from sticking together.

You can also find linoleic acid in safflower, sunflower, and soybean oils. But don't go overboard. A high ratio of omega-6 fatty acids (like linoleic acid) to omega-3 fatty acids can cause all sorts of health problems, including headaches, arthritis, asthma, and arrhythmia.

Catch more fish. It's this simple – more fish means less risk of stroke. Just eating about an ounce of fish a day, or two filets a week, will slash your stroke risk in half. That's because the omega-3 fatty acids in fish keep blood clots from forming. Cold-water, fatty fish like anchovies, bluefish, herring, mackerel, mullet, salmon, sardines, sturgeon, trout, tuna, and whitefish are your best bets for omega-3. If you can't stomach seafood, you can also find some omega-3 in flaxseed, walnuts, and dark leafy greens such as collards, spinach, arugula, Swiss chard, and kale.

Opt for olive oil. Rich in monounsaturated fat and vitamin E, this tasty oil decreases your blood's stickiness so it's less likely to clot. This lowers your blood pressure and reduces your risk for stroke.

Use olive oil for cooking and in salad dressings. But, as with any oil, don't go overboard. Oils weigh in at a hefty 120 calories a tablespoon.

Factor in tomatoes. Researchers at Scotland's Rowett Research Institute recently discovered that the yellow jelly around the seeds of a tomato has the power to prevent blood clots. Called "tomato factor," the jelly stops your blood's platelets from clumping together.

"Anti-platelet therapy in the form of aspirin is already routine in patients with some conditions. However, aspirin has side effects which can cause stomach upsets and bleeding," says Asim Dutta-Roy, senior scientist at the institute.

"Other anti-platelet drugs are also available but they can be expensive, and they are not used at an early stage to protect against cardiovascular disease. Finding a safe anti-platelet therapy that can be used to both prevent and treat these problems is, therefore, a priority." Strawberries, melons, and grapefruit also contain this potentially helpful substance.

Welcome wasabi. This popular sushi condiment, known as "Japanese horseradish," contains compounds called isothiocyanates which stop your platelets from clumping. The wasabi plant belongs to the cruciferous family, which also includes broccoli and cabbage.

Fill up on fruits and veggies. Looking to surprise your taste buds with something out of the ordinary? Try some eggplant and kale. These two vegetables contain substances that prevent blood from clotting, causing a stroke or heart attack.

They're called flavonoids, and you can find them in tea, red wine, onions, and a variety of fruits and vegetables. Some good sources include strawberries, grapefruit, apples, ginger, garlic, oregano, and black pepper.

Whatever the reason, fruits and vegetables have repeatedly been shown to lower your risk for stroke. One study found that cruciferous and green leafy vegetables and citrus fruit and juice provide the most protection.

Great ways to cook greens

Forget the fatback. Lose the lard. Give up on grease. Greens – such as spinach, Swiss chard, kale, collard, mustard, and turnip greens – can protect you from stroke, but not when they're greasy and fattening.

Here are some healthier ways to prepare greens.

- Blanch fresh greens in boiling water for several minutes, then drain and chop. Saute the greens with garlic, onions, and a little bit of olive oil until tender. This makes a scrumptious side dish.

- Wilt fresh greens in a covered saucepan and add sauteed mushrooms, onions, and garlic. Serve over pasta or a baked potato for an excellent entree.

- Thaw frozen greens in boiling water, then add them to your usual vegetable soup during the last five minutes of cooking to create a super soup.

Get creative with greens. Raw greens can spruce up a salad, while steamed or microwaved greens stay crisp and taste great.

Look for fresh greens at farmers' markets or grocery stores. They should have firm stalks and must be washed before cooking. Keep in mind that fresh greens can cook down to about a quarter of their original volume.

Essential vitamins you might be missing

You know vitamins play an important role in your overall health. Some even guard you from stroke. But don't stock your medicine cabinet with bottles of pills. You can find the vitamins you need in fruits, vegetables, and other delicious foods.

Vitamin C. This antioxidant vitamin gets an "A" for its ability to prevent stroke. It neutralizes free radicals, lowers blood pressure, strengthens blood vessel walls, and helps build collagen.

No wonder low levels of vitamin C mean a higher stroke risk. In a recent Finnish study, men with the lowest vitamin C levels (equal to half a glass of orange juice) were more than twice as likely to have a stroke as those with the highest.

> To get more vitamin C, eat the recommended five fruits and vegetables a day. These tasty foods are a healthier, cheaper and safer alternative to supplements.

If the men were overweight or had high blood pressure, their risk was even greater. This supported an earlier, 20-year Japanese study. In that study of 880 men and 1,241 women, those with the highest levels of vitamin C in their blood were 41 percent less likely to have a stroke as those with the lowest. Vitamin C-rich foods include sweet red peppers, strawberries, cantaloupe, brussels sprouts, grapefruit, oranges, lemons, limes, broccoli, green peppers, orange juice, tomato juice, and cabbage.

Vitamin E. This antioxidant also features anti-clotting powers. Not only does it lower cholesterol by preventing LDL oxidation, it also makes your blood less sticky so it's less likely to clot.

A preliminary Finnish study suggests vitamin E lowers the risk of stroke in men with high blood pressure. But other studies found no benefit from vitamin E supplementation. Food sources of vitamin E include wheat germ, vegetable oils, dark leafy greens, nuts, and seeds.

B vitamins. In a new Swiss study, people who recently underwent an angioplasty to clear their blocked arteries were given either a combination of B vitamins or a placebo. Those who took the B vitamins – folate, B12, and B6 – fared much better. This group needed significantly fewer repeat angioplasties and also suffered fewer heart attacks and deaths.

The homocysteine-lowering effect of folate probably helped. Homocysteine is a dangerous substance that encourages blood clots and hardening of the arteries. But vitamin B6's ability to stop platelets from clumping could have had something to do with it, too.

Studies often use supplements that give you more B vitamins than you get from your diet. But you can get plenty of these vitamins from foods. Here's where to look.

- Vitamin B6 can be found in dark leafy greens, seafood, legumes, whole grains, fruits, and vegetables.

- Vitamin B12 appears in meats, fish, dairy foods, and eggs.

- Folate can be found in dark leafy greens, legumes, seeds, and enriched breads and cereals.

Make an effort to get these helpful vitamins into your diet. After all, the right foods can keep your health from taking a wrong turn.

Recovery discoveries

Recovering from a stroke can be difficult. Fortunately, scientists are finding new tools to help.

Botox, known for its anti-wrinkle powers, also helps stroke victims who suffer from spasticity, or muscle tightness, in their wrists or fingers.

A recent study found that botox injections reduced pain and made everyday tasks, such as personal hygiene and dressing, much easier.

Another possible treatment is inosine, a chemical that helps your brain partially rewire itself after an injury. In a recent study of rats, researchers pumped either inosine or a saline solution into their brains after they had a stroke.

The inosine treatment:

- Helped rats sprout three times as many new connections from the undamaged side of the brain to the spinal cord. These helped replace the damaged links.

- Helped rats regain much more movement and perform tasks such as moving their legs, swimming, and retrieving some food.

- Was effective even up to 24 hours after a stroke.

These results show promise for humans, but research is still in its early stages. Keep your eyes and ears open for the latest developments.

Lower your risk with this amazing mineral

Cab Calloway playfully sang, "Have a banana, Hannah" in his 1947 song "Everybody Eats When They Come to My House." Hannah would have been wise to take him up on his offer. After all, bananas provide potassium, one of the most valuable weapons against stroke. Discover how potassium – as well as some other nutrients – can help you avoid a "brain attack."

Slash stroke risk. Potassium helps keep your blood pressure under control, especially when you also limit your sodium intake. Lower blood pressure means lower stroke risk. But potassium's powers go beyond its effect on blood pressure. Reduce your chance of having a stroke by up to 40 percent, simply by getting more of this natural mineral.

Boosting your potassium intake to 4 grams a day can help tremendously, according to a Harvard study. That would mean eating the equivalent of about nine bananas. If you're going bananas from eating bananas, get your potassium from leafy greens, broccoli, cantaloupe, oranges, potatoes, beans, milk, whole grains, meats, coffee, and tea.

Maximize your medication. If you take diuretics for high blood pressure, congestive heart failure, or kidney disease, make an effort to keep your potassium levels up. These medications, which remove water from your body, also get rid of potassium.

According to a recent study, diuretic users with the lowest levels of potassium in their blood were 2.5 times more likely to have a stroke than those with the highest levels.

"Diuretics clearly help prevent stroke by controlling high blood pressure," says Dr. Deborah Green of The Queen's Medical Center in Honolulu. "The question is whether diuretics would be even more effective with adequate potassium intake."

Provide extra protection. As powerful as potassium is, it could use a boost from some other anti-stroke nutrients. Make sure your diet also includes the following stroke stoppers.

- Fiber fights high cholesterol and high blood pressure, both risk factors for stroke. Eating 29 grams of fiber a day can drastically lower your stroke risk. If you have high blood pressure, adding just 10 grams of fiber to your diet every day can cut your risk of stroke by a whopping 41 percent. Cereal fiber, the kind in oats, wheat, rye, and barley, provides the most protection.

- Magnesium relaxes your blood vessels and balances the amount of potassium and sodium in your blood cells. Getting more than 450 mg of magnesium a day can significantly decrease your stroke risk. Good sources of magnesium include whole grain breads and cereals, broccoli, chard, spinach, okra, oysters, scallops, sea bass, mackerel, beans, nuts, and seeds. Also try avocado, black-eyed peas, almonds, squash, oatmeal, and baked potato with skin.

- Calcium, like potassium, helps get rid of sodium through your urine. You can find calcium in cheese, milk, yogurt, broccoli, spinach, turnip greens, mackerel, and salmon.

An easy way to boost your intake of potassium, magnesium, and fiber is to eat more fruits and vegetables. You'll enjoy a variety of delicious foods and guard against stroke at the same time. And that, unlike a Cab Calloway song, is no jive.

Healthy habits

Eating right, losing weight, and lowering your cholesterol and blood pressure certainly help – but your odds of avoiding a stroke can go up in smoke if you don't make some lifestyle changes.

- Stop smoking. This dangerous habit doubles your risk for having a stroke.
- Exercise regularly. Physical activity and fitness can markedly lower your chances of having a stroke.
- Deal with depression. Depression has been linked to stroke. See the *Depression* chapter for tips on coping or seek professional help.
- Avoid air pollution. A Korean study found a link between air pollution and stroke deaths. Heed smog alerts and limit trips outside on especially bad days.
- Think twice about chiropractic neck manipulation if you are at risk for stroke.
- Silence startling sounds. Loud noises or sudden movements can trigger a stroke. Muffle your doorbell and telephone and avoid sudden, jerky motions.
- Control your temper. Anger and other negative emotions often precede stroke.
- Get a flu shot. It may cut your risk for stroke in half.

CHAPTER 34 *Syndrome X*

What is Syndrome X? It's a potentially dangerous cluster of conditions centered around insulin resistance, an abnormality in the way your body's insulin metabolizes sugar. Also called insulin resistance syndrome, it can lead to heart disease and diabetes.

Who gets it? Experts estimate that one out of three Americans has it. Certain groups, like blacks, Latinos, Indians, and Asians, are more at risk. You're also more in danger if insulin resistance runs in your family, you're overweight, or you don't exercise.

What are the symptoms?

- high blood pressure
- low levels of "good" HDL cholesterol
- high levels of blood sugar, insulin, and triglycerides

You can overcome this 'silent killer'

Dr. Gerald Reaven is like the investment firm in those old television commercials. When he talks about Syndrome X, everybody listens.

Reaven is the Stanford University professor who first discovered and named Syndrome X. He recently published his findings from four decades of revolutionary research in the book *Syndrome X: The Silent Killer.*

At the heart of this work is an eating plan designed especially for Syndrome X sufferers. Follow it, and you may control your insulin, lower your low-density lipoprotein (LDL) cholesterol levels, and lose weight. Amazingly, you'll also find the plan easy, delicious, and nutritious.

Reaven's eating plan stands traditional medical wisdom on its head. For years, health experts recommended a low-fat, high-carbohydrate diet for a healthy heart. They believed carbohydrates should make up to 60 percent of your daily calories. That way, they'll replace saturated fats and keep your LDL cholesterol in check. But according to Reaven, all those carbohydrates can be disastrous if you have Syndrome X.

"It's so obvious," Reaven explains. "If you eat more carbohydrates, you need more insulin. And the more insulin resistant you are, the more insulin you need."

When you eat carbohydrates, your body breaks them down into simple sugars. Insulin's job is to wrangle up this sugar as it enters your bloodstream and lead it to your cells. The cells then take it up and use it for energy, and your blood sugar decreases. "Insulin acts to put carbohydrates in the right places," Reaven says.

If you have Syndrome X, however, your cells don't take in the sugar. Your body releases more and more insulin until, finally, the cells absorb the glucose, and your blood sugar drops. But the stress of all that insulin can damage the linings of your arteries and put you one step closer to heart disease.

Eat more "good" fat. Reaven's solution to this crisis may sound off-the-wall — trade in those extra carbohydrates for fat. It's not so crazy an idea, since it's the monounsaturated fatty acids (MUFAs) and polyunsaturated fatty acids (PUFAs) he's talking about. These are the "good" fats that don't increase your LDL cholesterol. And unlike carbohydrates, they won't raise your blood sugar.

Make these good fats 30 to 35 percent of your daily diet. Meanwhile, keep the unhealthy saturated fat to no more than 5 to 10 percent. "That accomplishes the same advantage for LDL cholesterol," Reaven states, "but it does it without the untoward effect of making you make more insulin."

To meet your daily ration of good fats, include sources of both polyunsaturated fatty acids and monounsaturated fatty acids. Fish, flaxseed and flaxseed oil, canola oil, walnuts, and seeds are all loaded with PUFAs. For MUFAs, try olive and canola oils, peanuts, almonds, cashews, pecans, and avocados. As for saturated fats, steer clear of red meat, whole-fat dairy products, eggs, coconut oil, and processed and fried foods.

Reverse the usual ratio of carbs.
Reaven's plan leaves carbohydrates as only 45 percent of your daily calories. Don't fret about the kind of carbohydrates. "Not as long as you're eating real food," suggests Reaven. Whole grains, fruits, and vegetables are all fine, as long as you maintain the 45-percent ratio.

> If you eat 2,000 calories a day, allow 900 calories for carbohydrates, 300 for protein, 600 to 700 for good fat, and not more than 100 to 200 for saturated fat.

Steady your protein intake. Believe it or not, protein can increase your insulin just like carbohydrates. So Reaven's plan keeps protein at a minimum – 15 percent of your calories. That might disappoint you if you're a fan of high-protein diets.

But considering the roller coaster ride these diets may send your blood sugar on, not to mention the saturated fat they usually contain, they may only make your insulin resistance, heart disease, and other symptoms of Syndrome X worse.

In the long-run, that could be fatal. Your pancreas, which is your body's insulin factory, could break down after years of pumping out too much of the hormone. That leaves you with Type 2 diabetes. Or you could be looking at a heart attack after all that damage to your blood vessels.

No wonder people listen when Reaven talks. If you want to follow his advice, work with your doctor to incorporate Reaven's guidelines into your own eating habits.

Calculate your risk

Carrying weight around your waist is a major risk factor for Syndrome X. To find out if your risk is high, try this easy, at-home test. It helps you gauge your waist-to-hip ratio in three simple steps.

- First, measure the smallest part of your waist with a tape measure. Be honest. No holding in your stomach!
- Size up your hips next, making sure to wrap the tape measure around the largest part of your buttocks.
- Divide your waist measurement by your hip measurement using a calculator.

For women, a result of 0.8 or higher means your abdomen is obese. And for men, a result of 1.0 or higher signals abdominal obesity.

Notify your doctor if you scored in the waist-to-hip danger zone. Then ask for a full Syndrome X workup. Your doctor will measure your glucose tolerance, triglycerides, high-density lipoprotein (HDL) cholesterol, blood pressure, and weight. This battery of tests can show for sure if you have the condition.

Lower your risk with milk

Tell the milkman to double your order. Dairy foods may prevent Syndrome X, according to researcher Mark A. Pereira and colleagues after they followed the diets of more than 3,000 people for 10 years.

Those who ate five or more dairy foods a day developed about two-thirds fewer cases of Syndrome X, compared with their peers who ate less than one-and-a-half servings a day.

Pereira and his fellow researchers suggested that dairy's rich supply of calcium, potassium, and magnesium could have something to do with it. These minerals are linked to lower rates of heart disease and Type 2 diabetes.

Unfortunately, only young adults were part of Pereira's study, and dairy foods seemed to help only those who were obese. Nevertheless, low-fat milk, yogurt, and cheese can be healthy additions to your daily menu – in moderation.

Healthy habits

"There are three major factors that regulate insulin resistance and how high your insulin is," says Dr. Gerald Reaven, the pioneer of Syndrome X research. "The major factor is genes. About half of it. The other half – about 25 percent of that – is fitness, and about 25 percent of it is fatness."

That means you have control over Syndrome X – if you follow these three lifestyle tips.

- Exercise at least 30 minutes every day. It's no surprise that men in a recent study who exercised more than three hours a week had half the risk of Syndrome X compared to men who rarely exercised.

- Plot out a weight loss plan with your doctor and follow it. "If you are insulin resistant and overweight," Reaven advises, "weight loss is going to make you more insulin sensitive." That means your body needs less of the hormone to lower your blood sugar. And less insulin means less harm to your heart and blood vessels.

- Quit smoking and limit your drinking. Smoking and excessive drinking can make Syndrome X worse.

CHAPTER 35

Ulcers

What are ulcers? They are sores in the lining of your stomach or the beginning of your small intestine.

Who gets them? Anybody can. One out of 10 Americans will have an ulcer in his lifetime.

What are the symptoms?

- weight loss
- poor appetite
- bloating, burping
- nausea or vomiting
- gnawing stomach pain that comes and goes for days or weeks at a time, occurs two to three hours after meals or in the middle of the night, and goes away when you eat or take an antacid

The best way to heal an ulcer

Ulcer sufferers used to have a hard life. They were trapped in strict diets, warned to avoid stress like the plague, and often blamed for their predicament. Fortunately, health experts now know differently. Being stressed out or eating spicy or acidic foods doesn't cause ulcers, but they can aggravate an ulcer you already have.

Most ulcers are caused by *Helicobacter pylori*, cork-shaped bacteria that burrow into your stomach's protective lining. This attack allows digestive acids to burn through the lining and cause the ulcer, or sore, in your stomach or small intestine.

Kill the *H. pylori* and, in most cases, you'll heal the ulcer. Antibiotics do the trick for most people. So visit your doctor if you suspect you have an ulcer. She can detect an *H. pylori* infection and prescribe medication to heal it.

> **If you can't give up spicy foods, don't. Show your doctor a list of your favorites and ask for a trial-and-error eating plan to determine which foods, if any, inflame your ulcer.**

In the meantime, search your kitchen for these natural healers. Some may soothe your stomach, while others could shield it from a bacterial attack. And some might even be *H. pylori* exterminators.

Cabbage. This member of the brassica plant family has long been a folk remedy for ulcers, and a recent study finally showed why. It's loaded with vitamins and plant compounds called phytochemicals, which protect your stomach's lining. Broccoli, broccoli sprouts, kohlrabi, brussels sprouts, and cauliflower – all members of cabbage's family tree – could be beneficial, too.

Cranberry juice. Health experts have known for years that cranberry juice fights urinary tract infections. This tart drink has its own type of phytochemicals that prevent bacteria from setting up shop.

Now researchers believe it might work against *H. pylori* in your stomach. One glass of cranberry juice a day could be enough to flush the bacteria out of your stomach – before they can dig in and wreak havoc.

Garlic. Next time you cook your favorite Italian dish, add plenty of this potent bacteria killer. In the laboratory, garlic extracts appeared to slow the growth of four different kinds of *H. pylori*.

Green tea. Reach for green tea when you're craving a warm drink and a little caffeine. Unlike black tea or coffee, green tea is gentler on your stomach. And drinking it regularly might help ease stomach inflammation.

Honey. Healers have used this golden delight for eons to fight infections. So it's no surprise today when scientists declare honey an ulcer healer. To help kill *H. pylori*, spread a tablespoon of honey on some bread and eat it an hour before meals and at bedtime. Don't drink anything with it so the honey will stay in your stomach long enough to work its healing magic.

Experts once believed only a special kind of New Zealand honey, called Manuka honey, had this special power. According to the latest findings, any unprocessed honey does the trick. Look for it at the grocery store or farmers' market.

> **Bees brew another stomach saver called propolis. This "mortar," used for building hives, eradicated *H. pylori* in laboratory studies. More research is needed to see if it works for people.**

Sweet potato. The spud's tastier and more colorful cousin packs a two-fisted punch against ulcers. Sweet potatoes are a great source of beta carotene, an antioxidant your body uses to make vitamin A. This vitamin protects your stomach lining and helps your stomach grow new cells.

And that's not all. Sweet potatoes are filled with fiber. Besides being a regular hero of your digestive system, fiber is especially protective in your stomach where it helps rebuild the lining.

Milk. Like cranberry juice, milk seems to flush bacteria from your stomach before they can cause problems. Plus, it's a great source of vitamin A, which protects your stomach from ulcer-causing invaders.

Yogurt. This dairy snack is a veritable bacterial zoo. As dangerous as this sounds, the "bugs" in yogurt are really the good kind that battle the bad kind, like *H. pylori*. What's more, yogurt can soothe your stomach when you take antibiotics to kill *H. pylori*.

When you feel that dull, gnawing pain coming on, reach for some yogurt. For best results, check the yogurt's label and make sure it says "active cultures." That means the good bacteria are inside, alive and kicking.

All of these foods can help your stomach when it's battling *H. pylori*. In some cases, however, there could be another explanation for your ulcer, such as nonsteroidal anti-inflammatory drugs (NSAIDs) or tumors. See your doctor to find the cause of your discomfort.

Another reason to treat Helicobacter pylori

You may have a vitamin B12 deficiency if you're infected with *H. pylori*. That's because this bacteria can interfere with how your body absorbs the nutrient.

In a study of 138 people with vitamin B12 deficiency, researchers found that more than half had *H. pylori*. When these people received medication that killed the bacteria, the deficiency vanished, too. This isn't surefire proof the bacteria interferes with vitamin B12 absorption, but it does suggest a strong link.

Here's how you can protect yourself:

• Bolster your diet with natural vitamin B12 sources, like tuna fish, clams, cottage cheese, beef, and chicken.

• Eat fortified cereals regularly. Tops on the list are General Mills Total, Kellogg's Special K, and Kellogg's All-Bran. All have 6 micrograms per serving, which is more than twice the daily recommended amount.

• Get tested for *H. pylori*. Your doctor will prescribe antibiotics if you're infected.

Left untreated, a vitamin B12 deficiency can lead to anemia, depression, nerve damage, muscle damage, and sometimes even paralysis.

Soothe your tummy with herbs

Herbal remedies have been popular for thousands of years, and now researchers know why. Herbs are great sources of powerful flavonoids and other antioxidants, compounds that sweep free radicals out of your body.

You probably already heard how free radicals can cause cancer, heart disease, and many other diseases. Now experts believe these rogue molecules may also have a role in forming ulcers.

"They may be a side effect of the inflammatory process," says Dr. Judith J. Petry, Medical Director of the Vermont Healing Tools Project. Free radicals are like pollution left behind when *Helicobacter pylori* bacteria attack your stomach. Then these scavenging free radicals irritate an already irritated ulcer.

By taking care of these free radicals, antioxidants may help heal your ulcer. "The antioxidant properties of botanicals as well as pharmaceuticals," Petry agrees, "are believed to contribute to their anti-ulcer effects."

Here's a short list of botanicals, or traditional herbal remedies, that are full of ulcer-fighting antioxidants.

Licorice. It's more than just candy. Licorice aids your stomach by battling free radicals, protecting the stomach lining, stopping *H. pylori* from spreading, and easing inflammation.

Your best bet is to buy supplements of deglycyrrhizinated licorice (DGL). They appear to offer all the benefits of licorice without the side effects. Herbalists recommend taking two to four chewable 380-milligram tablets, 20 to 30 minutes before meals for two to four weeks.

Angelica root. Besides protecting you with antioxidants, this herb also seems to reduce stomach acidity and rejuvenate the stomach lining. You can buy supplements at health food stores.

Just be sure to follow the dosage instructions, and avoid using this herb if you are taking blood thinners, like warfarin.

Caraway. Herbal experts know this tasty plant as a stomachic, which means a medicine that stimulates the actions of the stomach. To make a therapeutic tea, crush one to two teaspoonfuls of caraway seeds. Then pour about two-thirds of a cup of hot water over them. Drain after 10 to 15 minutes.

Lemon balm. This fragrant herb not only makes a delicious, soothing tea, it's a traditional remedy for stomach complaints and a potent bacteria killer. To make a warm bedtime drink, pour a cup of hot water over half an ounce of the herb. Strain after 10 minutes.

German chamomile. This flower is the latest fad in herbal medicine, and it lives up to its hype. It seems to reduce inflammation, fight bacterial infections, and boost your immune system. That's a great combination when you're fighting off an *H. pylori* infection.

To make chamomile tea, pour about two-thirds of a cup of boiling water over three teaspoons of the dried flower. Let it steep for five to 10 minutes before straining.

Bromelain. After analyzing the results of over 200 studies, researchers found this pineapple extract to be a possible ulcer blocker, as well as a first-rate anti-inflammatory and an excellent digestive aid. You can find bromelain supplements at your local pharmacy or health food store. Be sure to follow the dosage instructions closely.

Just remember – see your doctor before self-treating an ulcer with herbs. "Ulcers can be fatal if inadequately treated," Petry cautions. And since herbal supplements are not regulated in the United States, you could take bogus herbs and put yourself at risk without even knowing it. You really don't know if the product is what it says it is or not.

Exterminate 'bug' to protect eyes

Don't look now. *Helicobacter pylori* is at it again. This time the bacteria could attack your sight.

The stomach bug may have a role in glaucoma, the number two cause of blindness. In an eye-opening study from Greece, *H. pylori* infected nine out of 10 glaucoma sufferers. That's no coincidence.

Even more amazing, killing the bacteria with antibiotics appeared to reduce glaucoma symptoms and improve vision. Improvements are usually unheard of if you have this serious condition.

The researchers believe *H. pylori* can clog blood vessels in your eyes. This could cause eye pressure to build up, a major sign of glaucoma. If you treat the infection, the pressure seems to decrease.

Although more research needs to be done, the link looks promising. Exterminating *H. pylori* could be a cure for glaucoma, not just the symptoms. Keep your eyes peeled for the latest news.

Escape the menace of stomach cancer

Get rid of *Helicobacter pylori*, and you'll lower your risk of stomach cancer. Most people who get stomach cancer are infected with the bacteria. Yet, all hope is not lost, according to a Yale University study.

"Our results suggest," says researcher Susan Mayne, "that prevention strategies for these cancers should emphasize increased consumption of plant foods, decreased consumption of foods of animal origin with the possible exception of dairy products, and control of obesity."

So fill your plate with fruits, vegetables, whole grains, and legumes. The following foods are the most powerful stomach protectors around.

Broccoli sprouts. Some strains of *H. pylori* are strong enough to survive a battle with antibiotics. But they may not be able to escape from broccoli sprouts and their powerful disease-fighter, sulforaphane. In test-tube studies, this natural plant compound wiped out the toughest *H. pylori*.

"We showed that *Helicobacter pylori* strains resistant to multiple antibiotics were killed by sulforaphane in-vitro," reports Johns Hopkins researcher Jed W. Fahey. The substance also protects your stomach in other ways. "It boosts the body's own protective enzymes," he explains, "which could have both cancer preventive and antioxidant benefits."

Though more testing needs to be done, it can't hurt to nibble on some broccoli sprouts. Or try these other brassica vegetables – broccoli, cabbage, cauliflower, and brussels sprouts. They also contain sulforaphane.

Black beans. An innovative new study showed folate may stop mutations from occurring in your genetic material, or DNA. Otherwise, these mutations could lead to cancerous cells. The study was just a start, since the researchers were only giving folate supplements to dogs.

But don't wait to enjoy foods high in this important B vitamin. Just two cups of black beans can give you a day's supply. Other good sources include dark leafy greens, asparagus, avocado, green peas, seeds, and enriched breads and cereals.

Tea. Men who regularly drank tea during a 12-year study seemed to have half the risk of stomach cancer as men who didn't drink tea. The reason could be powerful antioxidants called polyphenols.

"This study provides direct evidence that tea polyphenols may act as chemopreventive agents against gastric and esophageal cancer development," suggests one of the researchers, Mimi C. Yu. Green tea seems to have the most polyphenols, with oolong and black tea close seconds.

Strawberries. These mighty morsels are packed with vitamin C. Not only can this nutrient kill *H. pylori*, it's also an antioxidant that sweeps away the free radicals left in the bacteria's wake. Plus, strawberries are a low-acid source of vitamin C, so they won't irritate your ulcer. Broccoli, cantaloupe, peppers, and brussels sprouts share this claim to fame.

Guava. It's also important to have a low-acid source of lycopene, the famed antioxidant and cancer fighter. Guava is a winner, as are papaya and watermelon. Tomatoes and pink grapefruit are better known sources of lycopene, but their acidity could upset your stomach.

Spinach. Learn a lesson from Popeye and eat more spinach. In a Korean study, researchers discovered that eating spinach and cabbage reduced the risk of stomach cancer, while eating broiled meats and salty foods increased the risk.

Herbs and spices. If you need another reason to give up salty foods, look no farther than these flavorful mealtime additions. Basil, rosemary, turmeric, ginger, and parsley add zing to any dish, as well as a hefty load of flavonoids and other powerful antioxidants. Herbal experts say fresh herbs are much more potent than the dried variety.

Onions. Half an onion a day keeps stomach cancer away. That's what Dutch researchers discovered in a study of more than 120,000 men and women. Making half an onion part of your daily menu could cut your risk of stomach cancer in half. Onions contain quercetin and other antioxidants that can safeguard your stomach.

Healthy habits

It's safe to smooch, according to the latest research. You can kiss your special someone without catching the dreaded *H. pylori* bacteria, experts say. But to prevent an ulcer flare-up, follow these tips.

- Eat fiber-rich and nutrient-packed foods, like fruits, vegetables, and whole grains.
- Space meals regularly throughout the day instead of just having snacks.
- Use caution with nonsteroidal anti-inflammatory drugs, also known as NSAIDs.
- Get a good night's sleep.
- Exercise regularly.
- Stop smoking.
- Learn to manage stress. Take up a new hobby or attend a yoga class.
- Practice moderation with stomach-irritating beverages, like coffee and alcohol.

CHAPTER 36

Urinary tract infections

What are urinary tract infections? They are serious health problems that start when bacteria attach to the outside of your urinary tract. They can spread up the urethra, the tube to your bladder, and reach your kidneys.

Who gets them? Women are most at risk. One out of five women suffers one in her lifetime. A kidney stone, an enlarged prostate, and diabetes increase your risk.

What are the symptoms?

- frequent urge to urinate
- burning, cloudy, milky, or even reddish urine
- sick feeling, tiredness, or shakiness
- pressure over your pubic bone, fullness in the rectum, or back pains

Surprising way to flush out bacteria

There's exciting news for millions of women and men. Scientists are busy developing a vaccine to prevent urinary tract infections (UTIs). But don't celebrate just yet. The Food and Drug Administration needs to perform more tests before they approve the vaccine. In the meantime, eat these foods to help keep your urinary tract healthy.

Citrus fruits. Oranges, lemons, grapefruit, and other citrus fruits are bursting with vitamin C. This multi-talented nutrient has its hands in everything from cancer protection to heart health, as well as UTI prevention. Eaten regularly, these fruits and their juices give you enough vitamin C to raise the acidity level of your urine. And that makes it an unfriendly place for bacteria to grow.

> Tired of guzzling cranberry juice? Try blueberries. Their flavonoids might prevent UTIs the same way — by stopping the bacteria from sticking to the walls of your urinary tract.

Cranberry juice. If you are prone to bladder infections, it's important to have a remedy that both prevents and treats them. Several studies have shown that cranberry juice does just that. In a recent study, it put the kibosh on bladder infections in nearly three out of four people. This tangy drink contains compounds called flavonoids, which prevent bacteria from clinging to the walls of your urinary tract. Without their footholds, the bacteria get washed away before an infection starts. One to two cups of pure cranberry juice a day could be all it takes to keep your urinary tract healthy.

Parsley. This popular herb is a diuretic, which means it makes you urinate more. Going to the bathroom very often can be embarrassing and annoying, unless you're at risk for a UTI. Frequent urination is a benefit since it flushes out bacteria before they can set up shop. To top it off, the herb is a great source of vitamin C. Be adventurous and try the Middle Eastern delicacy tabbouleh when dining out, since it's packed with parsley. If you plan to use parsley in your cooking, learn the difference between the two main kinds. The frilly, fern-like variety is best used as a garnish. The "Italian" flat-leafed variety has a stronger flavor and is perfect for cooking.

How to deal with an irritated bladder

A chronic, painful condition called interstitial cystitis (IC) affects more than 700,000 people in the United States alone, and as many as 90 percent are women. While it shares many of the same symptoms of a urinary tract infection (UTI) – bladder pain and frequent, intense urges to urinate – there's no infection. Instead, your bladder is irritated and scarred with bleeding sores the size of a pinhole.

Doctors have no easy answers for IC, since they're not even sure what causes it. Although antibiotics, cranberry juice, and other UTI remedies are powerless, many people are helped by the following suggestions:

Stay away from trigger foods. Spicy or acidic foods may irritate your bladder more. They include tomato-based foods, chocolate, caffeinated beverages, and citrus fruits. Alcohol and artificial sweeteners may have the same effect. Talk with your doctor about setting up an elimination diet to discover which foods cause problems for you.

Find help at the pharmacy. Over-the-counter medicines, like Prelief, reduce food acidity, making it safe to eat the chili, spaghetti sauce, and salsa you love. Aspirin and ibuprofen can help relieve discomfort.

Train your bladder. Set certain times to urinate during the day and stick to them. Keep a bathroom journal to track how often and when you urinate.

Stay calm. Learn a relaxation technique to overcome the pain of IC. Gentle stretching exercises, such as yoga, or an alternative therapy called biofeedback could also help.

Quit smoking. Add one more reason to the list. Smoking can worsen IC symptoms, not to mention cause bladder cancer.

Healthy habits

"Everyone has the bacteria that can cause bladder infections," says urologist Dr. Carole Gordon. "So to prevent bladder infections, the best thing to do is to have good bladder habits."

- Eat a high-fiber diet for soft, easy-to-pass stools. Gordon recommends a daily fiber supplement, too.

- Drink six to eight 8-ounce glasses of water a day. Sports drinks and fruit drinks are fine, but it's important to drink more water.

- Limit coffee, tea, sodas, and acidic foods if you have a bladder infection. "It is the acidity of these products that is irritating to the bladder lining," notes Gordon.

- Don't be a "bladder holder," she warns. Urinate every two to three hours in the daytime. Empty your bladder completely each time.

- Wipe front to back, and get in the habit of using wet wipes after every bowel movement.

- Wash your genital area daily with soap and water.

- Wear "breathable" cotton underwear.

- Forgo perfumes, douches, and bubble baths that can dry genital skin.

- Use hypoallergenic pads and tampons.

- Clean your genital area before and after intercourse, and urinate afterward.

CHAPTER 37

Weight control

What is the difference between being overweight and being obese? You are overweight if you weigh more than the average person for your height. The extra weight can come from bone, muscle, or fat. Obesity is having a dangerously high proportion of body fat and is a risk factor for chronic conditions like diabetes and heart problems.

Who's more likely to gain extra weight? People who are sedentary, who eat more calories than they use, or those with a family history of obesity are more likely to carry too much weight.

Who's at greater risk for disease because of weight?

- men with a waist circumference over 40 inches
- women with a waist circumference over 35 inches

Discover the only diet you will ever need

There is only one diet that helps you drop pounds and keep them off – the diet for a lifetime.

The four most important rules of this diet are: don't eat more calories than your body can burn, eat more plant-based foods than meat-based, keep an eye on your portion sizes, and exercise daily.

Eat only what you can burn. Follow this advice and you may not have to worry about being overweight again! This is, essentially, a "Nothing Forbidden" diet plan anybody can follow. What it means is, you can have that slice of cheesecake but you have to burn those extra calories off or your body stores them as fat.

Once you get to your ideal weight, the only way to maintain it is to eat only as many calories as your body will burn in a day — 1800-2000 calories is about average.

> Diversity will keep you on your diet. So choose as many different kinds of foods as possible — especially natural foods.

Redistribute your calories. How you spend each day's allotment of calories is extremely important. The National Academy's Institute of Medicine (IOM) just set new guidelines for a balanced diet that are much more flexible and easy to follow. And since this healthy diet isn't as low on fat as you might think, you should be able to enjoy all your favorite foods, as long as you eat them in moderation. According to the IOM, divide your calories along these lines:

- 45-65 percent should come from carbohydrates — the main component of grains, fruits, and vegetables.

- 20-35 percent can come from fat. But keep your intake of saturated fats as low as possible.

- 10-35 percent of your calories should come from protein sources like meat, legumes, nuts, eggs, and dairy.

Most people find it hard to recognize the right proportion of protein to carbohydrates. The answer, however, is right before your eyes.

Get control of your portions. The American Institute of Cancer Research (AICR) recently published *The New American Plate*, which says eating right is all about portion and proportion. They explain an easy way to judge how much food is too much.

- Take a look at your plate next time you sit down to dinner. If you eat like most people, meat might take up over half your plate. According to Melanie Polk, RD, Director of Nutrition Education at the AICR, this needs to change. "Reverse the traditional American plate, and think of meat as a side dish or condiment rather than the main ingredient. Meat should only cover one-third or less of your plate."

- "Plant-based foods," Polk says, "like vegetables, fruits, whole grains, and beans should cover two-thirds or more of your plate."

Traditional Plate

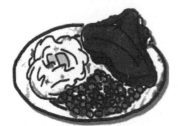

New American Plate

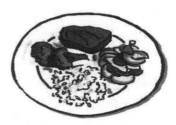

(Reprinted with permission from the American Institute for Cancer Research)

One way to switch to the new, healthier plate is to eat only half your usual portion of meat and have two vegetable sides instead of one. It's that simple.

Polk also notes that American serving sizes are far too big. In fact, obesity rates started climbing when restaurant portions tripled.

If you can't remember what a healthy portion should look like, there's an easy way to figure it out.

- Pull out two clean plates. On one, spoon out your usual portion of a food – for example, half a plate of noodles.

- Check the Nutrition Facts on the box of noodles and you'll discover a serving size is probably around half a cup.

- Now measure out half a cup – or one serving – of noodles and place it on the second clean plate.

You might be surprised how much smaller a single serving should be. "What we are recommending," says Polk, "is that if you weigh more than you would like to, or more than you should, take a look at your portion sizes and see how many standard serving sizes are included in those portions. Then start to cut down a little bit. This doesn't mean you have to cut out the food, it just means you may want to decrease the size of your portion."

Here are some sample servings sizes from the USDA.

Item	Serving size	Compare to
Whole vegetables and fruit	One medium vegetable or piece of fruit	A baseball
Chopped vegetables and fruit	1/2 cup	A rounded handful
Meat	3 ounces	A deck of cards
Rice, mashed potatoes, or pasta	1/2 cup cooked	A tennis ball
Snacks (nuts or pretzels)	1/3 cup	A level handful
Cheese	1 1/2 to 2 ounces	4 dice

Remember, according to the USDA Food Pyramid, you need three to five servings a day of both fruits and vegetables, and seven to 11 of grains.

Work your body. The crowning jewel of any healthy diet is exercise. The IOM recommends you exercise moderately for an hour every day. That's double the amount previously recommended by many experts. But exercise doesn't have to be done on a treadmill — you can climb stairs, take a walk, or do water aerobics. Even working hard at your chores counts.

Follow this program and you will lose pounds and keep them off forever.

Fight fat with water and fiber

Hunger pangs are a dieter's worst enemy. The perfect solution is to eat, feel full, and not gain an ounce. If this sounds too good to be true, welcome to the world of energy dense foods.

Add water and cut fat. Energy density is just a fancy way to say a food has a certain amount of calories, or energy, per unit of weight. Two ingredients affect energy density the most — water and fat.

Water has no calories, or zero energy density, so generally, the higher the water content, the lower the energy density of a food. And fat packs a lot of calories in every ounce, so the higher the fat content of a food, the higher the energy density.

> **Heavier people tend to eat more high-density foods like meat, butter, cheese, and sweets. People who are thinner often fill up on low-density foods like beans, grains, fruits, and vegetables.**

For example, you can make both chicken soup and chicken casserole with the same ingredients.But since chicken soup has more water, it is less energy dense. Therefore, you'll take in fewer calories to feel full. The high-density casserole, on the other hand, packs in a lot of calories in a relatively small serving. So you'll be getting more calories in order to feel full.

Fill up on fiber. Low-density foods are often high in fiber as well as water. This combination swells in your stomach, turning off your body's internal hunger switch. As an added bonus, fiber breaks down very slowly so you feel full for hours and can eliminate snacks. That's why fiber is often called the #1 weight-loss food.

One of the easiest ways to lower the energy density of a meal is to add whole grains, beans, fruits, and vegetables. Not only are they low-calorie, they're also full of nutrients that lower your cholesterol and blood pressure.

- **Whole grains.** Those grains that are as close to their natural form as possible are more likely to be low-energy dense foods. Switch to whole-wheat bread and pasta, and stay away from refined flours. Comfort foods like porridge and oatmeal are also a dieter's best friend. They fill you up for hours and dampen the constant cravings that keep you from losing the weight you want to lose.

- **Beans.** Known as the 50¢ meal, beans are the cheapest and best source of fiber. Not only that but these nutritious legumes are also low-calorie and full of protein. In fact in one study, a group of healthy men didn't cut calories but added about two and a half cups of beans to their usual daily menu. They still lost weight.

  Beans also lower your bad cholesterol, contain anti-cancerous agents, and relieve constipation.

  You can easily add beans to your diet by tossing them into every soup recipe, mixing them into your salads, and topping potatoes with chili instead of butter and cheese.

- **Fruits and vegetables.** The recommended daily amount of fiber for seniors is 30 grams for men and 21 grams for women. Eat an apple and you're 4 grams closer to that goal. Other fiber-rich fruits include raspberries, blackberries, pears, prunes, and dried figs. Among veggies, choose broccoli, sundried tomatoes, okra, potatoes (with skin), squash, and turnip greens.

You don't have to be a health nut to get enough fiber from plant foods. Just add a cup of veggies to your pasta, stir-fry some with chicken, or add fruit to your desserts and salads.

Foods rich in fiber and water can help you lose weight and keep it off. But add fiber slowly to your diet – too much too fast and you might get bloated and gassy. At the same time, don't completely write off high-density foods. Your body needs the nutrients in meat, dairy, and oils for many of its functions. Instead, focus on eating mostly low-density foods and add high-density foods in moderation.

Top 10 healthy eating tips

Here are some fun and easy ways to lose weight permanently and lower your blood pressure at the same time.

- Set realistic goals. Expect to lose 10 percent of your weight. Reward yourself for reaching mini-goals.
- Keep a food diary. Write down what you eat and how you feel.
- Create a weekly food plan and leave room for the occasional treat.
- Cook your own meals to control your portion size, fat content, and nutrients.
- Eat five small meals a day. This may keep you from unhealthy snacks.
- Start your day with fiber-rich whole grains and fruit.
- Drizzle a little olive oil on your greens.
- Drink orange juice a half-hour to hour before each meal. A Yale University researcher says this nutrient-loaded beverage helps you eat fewer calories.
- Sit down and savor your food. Always stop eating when you feel full.

- Turn up the lights. You may be less likely to overeat if you can see your food.

Calculate your health risks

There are two easy ways to tell if your weight might affect your health.

Measure your waist. The National Heart, Lung, and Blood Institute suggests you take a simple waist measurement to assess your risk of developing heart disease and type 2 diabetes. Wrap a measuring tape snugly around the widest part of your middle. If you are a man with a waist measurement over 40 inches, or a woman measuring over 35 inches, you are at risk – it's time to lose some abdominal fat.

Calculate your BMI. The Body Mass Index (BMI) is a comparison of your height to your weight. A healthy BMI is anywhere from 18.5 to 24.9. If your BMI is below 18.5 you are considered underweight. If your BMI is 25 to 29.9, you are slightly overweight – which carries some health risk. But if your BMI is 30 or over, talk to your doctor about weight loss programs since you are considered obese.

Obesity increases your risk of many chronic diseases – like diabetes, cancer, and stroke – and it's uncomfortable to live with. The good news is that losing just a few pounds can dramatically reduce these risks, and put you in a healthier BMI bracket.

Gain as you grey. Researchers at the Yale University School of Medicine believe seniors should live by a slightly different set of BMI guidelines. They say restricting calories – and therefore energy – if you are moderately overweight and 65 or older can have negative health effects.

According to study results from more than a dozen trials, these experts say you aren't considered at risk until your BMI tops 27. Gaining some weight at this age is natural and healthy. In fact, losing weight unnecessarily – as little as 5 percent of your body weight – can increase your risk of dying by 67 percent. So consult your doctor before jumping on the diet bandwagon.

Body Mass Index (BMI) for general population

Weight	100	110	120	130	140	150	160	170	180	190	200
Height											
5'0"	20	21	23	25	27	29	31	33	35	37	39
5'1"	19	21	23	25	26	28	30	32	34	36	38
5'2"	18	20	22	24	26	27	29	31	33	35	37
5'3"	18	19	21	23	25	27	28	30	32	34	35
5'4"	17	19	21	22	24	26	27	29	31	33	34
5'5"	17	18	20	22	23	25	27	28	30	32	33
5'6"	16	18	19	21	23	24	26	27	29	31	32
5'7"	16	17	19	20	22	23	25	27	28	30	31
5'8"	15	17	18	20	21	23	24	26	27	29	30
5'9"	15	16	18	19	21	22	24	25	27	28	30
5'10"	14	16	17	19	20	22	23	24	26	27	29
5'11"	14	15	17	18	20	21	22	24	25	26	28
6'0"	14	15	16	18	19	20	22	23	24	26	27
6'1"	13	15	16	17	18	20	21	22	24	25	26
6'2"	13	14	15	17	18	19	21	22	23	24	26
6'3"	12	14	15	16	17	19	20	21	22	24	25

Should you moo shu?

Ethnic restaurants can have baffling menus. To figure out which dishes won't add to your weight, look for these menu tip-offs.

- **Italian.** Stay away from Alfredo, carbonara, parmigiana, and anything that's stuffed or fried. Choose entrees described as primavera, piccata, marinara, grilled, or thin crust.

- **Chinese.** Crispy, crunchy, sweet and sour, and fried dishes are all loaded with calories. Look for steamed dishes and ones containing these words: jum, kow, and shu.

- **Mexican.** Eat nachos, chimichangas, guacamole, and taco salad shells only rarely. Fill up on fajitas, entrees with shredded meat, soft corn tortillas, salsa, rice or black beans.

- **French.** Lovely as they are, limit entrees with these words: pâté, crème, au gratin, fromage, hollandaise, en croute, béarnaise, mousse, foie gras, or pastry. Instead, enjoy the delicate flavor of fruit sauces and choose poached, roasted, or en papillote dishes.

- **Indian, Thai, and Island fare.** Limit the amount of fritters and coconut dishes, and indulge in marinated, steamed, stir-fried, tandoori, Tikka, and satay dishes.

Avoid fast food pitfalls

Let's face it – it's almost impossible to dodge the drive-thru. But eating super-sized and deep-fried will play havoc with your diet. So here are some handy tips for the next time you must have fast food.

- Never, ever super-size a meal.

- Order a small or regular size burger instead of the quarter-pounder with cheese. You'll cut 250 calories.

- Skip the large fries and save 540 calories. That's about the calorie equivalent of an entire meal.

- Think grilled when choosing chicken or fish. Frying can cost you over 100 calories.

- Call in a thin crust veggie pizza. It's not only more nutritious, it's also a calorie bargain. Compare its 190 calories per slice to the 470 calories you get from one slice of stuffed-crust meat-lover's pizza.

- Order the taco salad but don't eat that deep-fried taco shell. You'll shave 370 calories off your dinner tab.

- Ask for a separate take-out box as soon as you place your order. Then split your meal in half when you get it and box it up for later.

- Choose your condiments wisely. Mustard has just 3 calories in one teaspoon, while mayonnaise has 19. And remember a teaspoon is not much – about the amount in one fast food packet. Most people use much more.

- Green salads are great ways to fill your vitamin bank. But trade the croutons and Parmesan cheese for seeds, nuts, and vegetable toppings.

- Shun the creamy salad dressings and go for a vinaigrette. Ask for your dressing on the side, and use only half of it.

- Select vegetable sides instead of pasta salads at the buffet. Not only are they more nutritious, they can carry about 100 to 300 fewer calories.

- Stop after just one meat serving or calorie-laden side dish at the all-you-can-eat buffet. Try a bowl of soup instead.

- Order water with lemon instead of a regular carbonated drink. You won't even notice the 120 to 150 calories you save with every glass.

Consider unusual causes of weight gain

Eating too much food is not always the reason behind your weight gain. Though relatively rare, there are three other causes you might want to ask your doctor about.

- **Thyroid problems.** Your thyroid controls how fast you use energy. If it produces too little thyroid hormone (a condition called hypothyroidism), you can gain weight. Ask your doctor for a simple blood test if you regularly feel cold and fatigued.

- **Heredity.** Genetics can play a strong role in weight gain. You could have too little of the hormone that signals you are full, or a speedy metabolism that processes fat a little too efficiently, which means you store it away like a squirrel before winter.

- **Medications.** Weight gain can be a side effect of some anti-depressants and estrogen, as well as of drugs used to treat blood pressure and diabetes — among many other conditions. Don't stop taking your meds. Share your concerns about your weight with your doctor. He may recommend a similar drug without this side effect.

Get milk and get slim

Can you drink milk and lose weight? New research shows adding calcium to your diet can help you lose body fat.

Dr. Robert Heaney, with the Osteoporosis Research Center of Creighton University, found that women with low calcium levels were more than twice as likely to be overweight. Then, in a group of 780 dieters, those who got the most calcium lost more weight than those without extra calcium. And perhaps more importantly, other research indicates a calcium-rich diet means you'll lose body fat, not lean muscle.

Animal research at the University of Tennessee, conducted by Dr. Michael Zemel, discovered that a low-calorie, high-dairy diet caused a loss of up to 70 percent of body fat. Low-calorie, low-calcium diets only reduced fat by 8 percent.

Both Zemel and Heaney think that calcium helps control how you burn fat. When your calcium levels are low, your body thinks you're starving, so it stores fat. When they are high, it burns fat more efficiently. So, in other words, you can raise your metabolism and drop pounds with calcium.

Bump up your numbers. More than half of all adults in the U.S. don't get the recommended amount of calcium – which the National Academy of Sciences has set at 1,000 to 1,200 milligrams (mg) a day for seniors. But just adding one to two serving of dairy (from 300 to 600 mg of calcium) to your diet every day, can make a difference in your weight.

> **Cream cheese, sour cream, coffee creamer, and whipping cream or other whipped topping contain little or no calcium.**

Watch the fat. Remember though that calcium is no magic diet pill. It only helps you lose weight if you're already on a reduced-calorie diet. So add calcium-rich dairy to your meals only if you cut calories somewhere else.

According to the Virginia Cooperative Extension Service, here are some calcium choices that, as you can see, vary greatly in their fat content.

Calcium (mg)	Low-fat food choice	Fat (g)	Medium-fat food choice	Fat (g)	High-fat food choice	Fat (g)
300	1 cup skim milk	0	1 cup whole milk	8	1 cup eggnog	19
200	1 oz low-fat cheese	6	1 oz American cheese	9	1/8 of 8" Quiche Lorraine	39
100	4" pan-cake	4	7" waffle	11	1 cup com-mercial granola	20

Dig into dairy. Here are some easy ways to include dairy foods in a low-calorie diet.

- Add low-fat milk to your coffee and tea.

- Cook warm cereals with low-fat milk instead of water.

- Substitute a smoothie blended with fruit, ice, and low-fat milk for that high-calorie milk shake.

- Treat yourself to half a cup of low-fat frozen yogurt.

- Add two servings of low-fat yogurt to your daily menu. Mix in some fruit for a yummy desert.

- Bake with milk instead of water (except yeast breads).

- Sprinkle fat-free dry milk powder on almost anything. You won't notice the taste or calories, and 2 tablespoons add about 100 extra milligrams of calcium.

Hunt down other sources. If you're lactose intolerant or don't like milk, you can still beef up on calcium without dairy.

- While calcium supplements are only about half as effective as dairy in helping you lose weight, you can try a daily dose of around 500 mg of calcium citrate.

- Canned sardines and salmon with bones are calcium-rich. So are dark green vegetables, like collards, turnip greens, kale, broccoli, rutabagas, and Chinese cabbage. Spinach has calcium, but your body can't absorb it.

- Some packaged foods also have added calcium. Fortified orange juice can have almost as much calcium as milk. Enriched cereals, soy-based foods, canned tomatoes, and stone ground flour can all have calcium added during processing. Read nutrition labels for your best sources.

Keep in mind that calcium is only a small piece of the big diet puzzle. It can help your body lose weight, but not on its own.

Popular diets: what works, what doesn't

From diets featuring peanut butter to ice cream, there seems to be a weight loss strategy for every taste. But before you jump on the latest bandwagon, see how your diet rates against this standard.

- For a diet to work, you must eat fewer calories than you burn.

- Your food choices should provide all the vitamins, minerals, and other nutrients you need to stay healthy.

- A successful diet will be diverse, so you never get bored and give up.

Here's how some of today's most popular diets stack up.

High-protein/low-carb diets. Eating plans, similar to the Atkins diet, recommend you cut carbohydrates without restricting fat or protein. Presumably your body burns more fat when it isn't supplied with a steady stream of easy carbohydrates to burn.

Recent short-term studies show some people lose more weight on this diet than on a low-fat diet. And surprisingly, this eating plan can also lower your cholesterol.

But before you banish carbohydrates, remember your diet must provide all the nutrients you need. When you limit vegetables, fruit, and grains, you put your health at risk.

In addition, a high-protein diet usually means more saturated fat – which can block your arteries – and an overabundance of ketones – waste products from protein and fat. A buildup of ketones in your blood, called ketosis, can increase production of uric acid, a risk factor for gout and kidney stones. This condition is especially risky for people with diabetes.

Until there are more long-term studies, get your doctor's approval and supervision before you begin this diet.

If you're a woman who's suffered from depression, don't diet too strictly. Going very low-cal can keep your body from producing enough serotonin — a mood hormone that helps keep you happy.

Low-fat diets. Eating plans like the Dean Ornish Life Choice Program stress an almost vegetarian lifestyle, with only 10 percent of your calories coming from fats. Ornish suggests that your body was designed to function best on a diet of mostly plant-based foods. It stores fat – or energy – for later, when you might need it. If you cut out fat, and eat a varied diet of fruit, vegetables, whole grains, and beans, you will fill up faster and speed up your metabolism.

Along with diet, Ornish also encourages you to exercise, manage stress, and stay connected to friends and family. He says you can not only lose weight, but also reverse the effects of heart disease.

Keep in mind this diet is pretty strict. You might have a hard time cutting meat and fats (including olive oil) and avoiding sugar and salt. Getting enough fresh, unprocessed foods will undoubtedly be a challenge for many people in today's fast-paced society.

You'll also need to watch your nutrient intake to make sure you don't become deficient in vitamins E, B12, and D, as well as calcium. However, if you eat a variety of vegetarian protein sources — like rice plus beans — you should meet your body's amino acid requirements.

Medium-fat diets. These diets loosely follow the eating habits of Mediterranean cultures — Greeks, southern French, and some Italians, for example — who usually get over 30 percent of their calories from fat. But not just any fat — they eat "good" monounsaturated fat from olive oil and nuts, and get less saturated fat. The Mediterranean diet also recommends fish, fruits, vegetables, and beans, and using whole grains and yogurt freely.

This eating plan may be the perfect balance between the low-fat and high-protein diets. It's diverse and flavorful enough to keep you on the diet, but it cuts back on harmful fats and refined grains. It also lines up with official health organizations' recommendations for acceptable intakes of fat and carbohydrates.

Prepared meal plans. These programs deliver pre-cooked balanced meals — usually low-fat and low-calorie — directly to your door. Research shows this approach can work, resulting in weight loss, improved heart health, and perhaps most importantly, an improved quality of life.

Liquid and supplement diets. Replacing one to three meals a day with just a shake can be a hard regimen to stick to. But research shows if you're diligent it can work — even over the long-term. This kind of diet seems especially beneficial to people who simply cannot change their eating habits. Controlling your food intake for even one meal is a daily reminder not to overeat.

Food points systems. Diets like Weight Watchers assign points to every food, based on fat, fiber, and calorie content. You pick and choose what you want to eat as long as you stay within a certain number of points every day. For motivation, you can join a weekly accountability group that keeps you on track. This diet can work as long as you don't cut out foods with good nutrients just because they have high point values.

Fad diets. Diets that promise fast and major weight loss often sound too good to be true – that's because they are. Be wary of any diet that is trying to sell a product, that is based on testimonials instead of solid research, or excludes whole categories of food. Remember too, that many natural or herbal weight loss products are not reviewed or given approval by the U.S. Food and Drug Administration (FDA).

This organization recommends you plan to lose just one to two pounds a week on any diet. Your best bet is to eat 300 to 500 fewer calories every day and exercise regularly – a winning recipe for steady, permanent weight loss.

Think *before* you fast

If you're considering a quick detox diet, you may reconsider when you learn what happens to your body when you fast.

- The dramatic weight you lose at first is just water.
- Soon you're burning fat – but also muscle.
- Substances like ketones collect in your body and your mineral levels drop. Among other things, this could cause severe heart problems.

- Your metabolism slows – you burn less fat – and other body processes slow or stop completely.

When you stop fasting, it's likely you will gain weight back quickly – and most of it will come back as fat and water. A long fast can also permanently damage your heart and weaken your immune system.

Don't endanger your health just to lose a few pounds. If you must, fast for no more than 24 hours and drink plenty of water to stay hydrated.

Outsmart sugar cravings with super snacks

Sugar cravings can derail even the most carefully planned diet. But if you substitute these healthy munchies for sweet heavy-hitters you can snack yourself thin.

- Chew sugar-free gum and burn 20 percent more calories.

- Eat an apple or a handful of baby carrots between meals. Naturally sweet, they can tide you over to the next meal.

- Add protein, like cottage cheese or peanut butter, to your snack to feel full longer.

- Substitute beverages like black or green tea for sugary sodas. According to one popular story, switching to tea as your only beverage may help you drop the pounds. The caffeine is thought to speed up your metabolism, helping you burn fat faster.

- Reach for peanuts. Unlike most salty foods, peanuts will not make you crave sugar. They're protein-rich and very satisfying, and you'll compensate for the extra calories naturally.

- Air-pop your own popcorn and flavor it with spices. This is a fiber-rich, low-cal alternative to sweets.

- Measure out a handful of unsalted pretzels. They're lower in fat than many other snacks.

- Savor one piece of hard or chewy candy a bit before a meal. The sugar rush should hit in time to help you eat less.

- Don't grab cookies. Keep some crunchy vegetables cut up in the fridge. Some diets say eating celery, cucumbers, and iceberg lettuce can burn more calories than they create. Whether you call them low-calorie or negative-calorie, these healthy bites are good weight-loss bets.

Rank your carbs to get thin

The concept of the Glycemic Index (GI) has been around for 20 years. Most people still don't understand it or know how to use it. But now, Harvard University introduces the concept of Glycemic Load (GL) – a clearer way to classify carbohydrates and their effect on your weight.

Your body burns sugar like your car burns gas, and carbohydrates are your main source of this fuel. Different carbs break down into glucose – or sugar – at different rates, depending on their structure. Some burn quickly in jagged peaks of energy, while some follow a gentler curve and break down slowly.

Carbohydrates signal your body to produce insulin, a hormone that controls how you metabolize food – including whether or not you store fat in your body. When you eat a lot of quick-burning carbs your blood sugar and insulin levels spike. This, ultimately, encourages your body to store fat. Slow-burning carbs, on the other hand, keep your insulin, your blood sugar, and your appetite steady.

Glycemic Index. According to experts backing the concept of the GI, every food can be ranked – from 0 to 100 – based on how much it will raise your blood sugar level.

Researchers always test a portion of food equal to 50 grams of carbohydrates. For example, that would be 200 grams of spaghetti, three and one-half slices of sandwich bread, or 60 grams of jelly beans. This way, as the saying goes, experts are comparing apples to apples.

Then, they measure the average amount of glucose in your system within two hours of eating this standard portion. The end result is a number they call the Glycemic Index (GI) of that food.

They believe the higher the GI, the bigger the insulin spike, the faster you feel hungry, and the more fat you store.

The Glycemic Index sounds like it could be a great weight-control tool, except for a few glitches that make it difficult for ordinary people to apply the concept in real life.

- Ripeness of fruit affects its GI.

- How a food is prepared affects its GI. For example, mashed potatoes differ from baked potatoes. Thick linguini has a lower GI than thin linguini.

- Eating a combination of carbohydrates, protein, and fat will influence the GI of that meal.

- Since the GI will vary greatly from food to food, you must refer to a standard list in order to make precise food choices.

- The Glycemic Index does not depend on a serving size, yet this greatly influences a food's effect on your blood sugar.

Glycemic Load. Because of these and other problems, researchers refined the idea and came up with Glycemic Load (GL). This takes the GI and applies it to a specific portion of that food. GLs are generally lower than GIs.

You can estimate a food's Glycemic Load by multiplying its Glycemic Index (with glucose as the reference food) by the amount of carbohydrate contained in a specific serving size, then dividing by 100.

Unless you are diabetic, keeping track of GLs while you shop may be more trouble than it's worth. However, to avoid gaining weight from insulin spikes, here are some basic GL guidelines to help you make better food choices.

- Resist the obvious – potatoes and foods with added sugar are fast burning carbs.

- Choose whole-grain, less processed foods over refined grain products. Stone-ground breads and old-fashioned oatmeal are better choices.

- Beans have very low GLs and are full of healthy fiber – a good bet for any meal.

- Most fruits and vegetables have low GLs. Very few – like corn, dried fruits, and bananas – have higher numbers than you might expect.

The beauty of low-GL foods is that they have fewer calories than high-protein or high-fat foods, and they're more satisfying.

Food	Type	Portion	GI*	GL
Bread	whole-grain	30g	51	7
Bread	white	30g	73	10
Potato	baked	150g	85	26
Macaroni	boiled	180g	45	22
White long-grain rice	boiled	150g	56	23
Brown rice	steamed	150g	55	18
Barley	boiled	150g	25	11
Apple	raw	120g	38	6

Apple juice	unsweetened	250ml	40	12
Orange	raw	120g	48	5
Orange juice	unsweetened	250ml	50	13
Carrots	raw	80g	16	1
Carrots	boiled	80g	92	5

*Glucose sugar was used as the reference food to determine the GI value.

For a reprint of a larger list of foods and their GI and GL numbers contact *The American Journal of Clinical Nutrition*:

- 9650 Rockville Pike, Bethesda, MD 20814-3998
- 301-530-7038
- www.ajcn.org

Healthy habits

Eating right is only half your ticket to great looks and good health. Being fit protects you from disease and defines how fast you lose weight. Here are some easy ways to get your body in gear.

- Follow a European tradition and take a walk after dinner. It will get those digestive juices going.
- Thump your feet. Tap your fingers. Fidgeting is a form of exercise that can burn an average of 348 calories a day.
- Buy a pedometer and walk 10,000 steps a day.
- Ask about mall-walking programs near you.
- Join a local hiking club. They usually have different age and difficulty levels to choose from.
- Learn new steps and meet new people at a dance class offered by your local recreation department.

- Make sleep a priority. Research indicates people snoozing less than six hours every night are more likely to be overweight.

Sources

Allergies

5 Years Without Food: The Food Allergy Survival Guide, Adapt Books, Louisville, Colo., 1997

Common Food Allergens, The Food Allergy and Anaphylaxis Network <www.foodallergy.org> retrieved Jan. 24, 2003

Environmental Health Perspectives (109,8:815)

Food Allergy and Intolerances, National Institute of Allergy and Infectious Diseases <www.niaid.nih.gov> retrieved Jan. 30, 2003

Gailen D. Marshall, Jr. M.D., Ph.D. Director of the Division of Allergy and Clinical Immunology, University of Texas Houston Medical School, Houston, Texas

Journal of Agricultural and Food Chemistry (50,20:5729)

Journal of Allergy and Clinical Immunology (107,2:367; 107,2:759)

New England Journal of Medicine (346,23:1833)

Pediatric Allergy and Immunology (11,2:71)

Primary Care; Clinics in Office Practice (29,2:231)

Statistics on Asthma and Allergic Diseases, American Academy of Allergy, Asthma and Immunology <www.aaaai.org> retrieved Jan. 21, 2003

The Complete Home Wellness Handbook, Rebus, Inc., New York, 2001

Your Hidden Food Allergies Are Making You Fat, Prima Health Publishing, Roseville, Calif., 1998

Alzheimer's disease

Alzheimer's Society press release (Oct. 21, 2002)

Archives of Neurology (59,2:223)

Atherosclerosis (161,2:293)

British Medical Journal (325,7370:932)

History of High Blood Pressure May Be Linked to Alzheimer's, Presented at: The International Conference on Alzheimer's Disease and Related Disorders; July 22, 2002; Stockholm, Sweden

International Journal of Geriatric Psychiatry (15,3:226)

Let's Go Nuts, Nutrition News <www.smudining.com> retrieved Oct. 23, 2002

Mayo Clinic Guide to Self-Care, Mayo Clinic, Rochester, Minn., 1999

Neurology (55,8:1158; 58,9:1333)

Nutrition in Clinical Care (4,3:140)

Proceedings of the National Academy of Sciences (98,6:3440)

Product Review: Ginkgo Biloba, Consumer labs <www.consumer lab.com> retrieved Sept. 6, 2000

Rush University news release (June 25, 2002)

Statin Use Is Associated with Reduced Risk of Alzheimer's Disease, Paper presented at: American Academy of Neurology's 54th

Annual Meeting, April 13-20, 2002, Denver, Colo.

Stroke (33,10:2351)

World Alzheimer Congress, July 9-18, 2000, Washington

Asthma

American Journal of Respiratory and Critical Care Medicine (165,9:1299)

Asthma and Older People, American Lung Association <www.lun gusa.org/asthma/astasthage.html> retrieved Feb. 10, 2003

British Medical Journal (320,7232:412)

Can Your Kitchen Pass the Food Safety Test? U.S. Food and Drug Administration <www.fda.gov/fdac/features/ 895_kitchen.html> retrieved Jan. 16, 2002

Cochrane Database of Systematic Reviews (2:CD001112)

Current Opinion in Allergy and Clinical Immunology (1:421)

Do Dietary Factors Protect Against Chronic Obstructive Pulmonary Disease: A Case Control Study, Poster presentation at: American Thoracic Society 97th International Conference; May 2001; San Francisco

Journal of Medicinal Food (3,2:115)

Journal of the American Pharmaceutical Association (40,6:785)

The Relationship of Respiratory Symptoms and Lung Function With Intakes of Apples and Tomatoes, Poster presentation at: American Thoracic Society 97th International Conference; May 2001; San Francisco

Thorax (55,2:102)

U.S. Pharmacist (25,7:42)

Atherosclerosis

Acute and Chronic Tea Consumption Reverses Endothelial Dysfunction in Patients with Coronary Artery Disease, Paper presented at: American Heart Association Scientific Sessions 2000; Nov. 13-16, 2000; New Orleans

Advances in Experimental Medicine and Biology (505:95)

American Journal of Cardiology (88,10:1139)

American Journal of Clinical Nutrition (75,5:880; 76,3:582; 76,6:1261)

American Journal of Epidemiology (149,2:162; 155,9:827)

American Journal of Medicine (112,7:535)

Archives of Internal Medicine (161,18:2185)

Arteriosclerosis, Thrombosis and Vascular Biology (21,10:E34)

Atherosclerosis (148,1:49)

Chemosphere (46,7:1053)

Circulation (103,14:1863; 103,22:2674; 103,24: 2922; 105,21:2476)

Current Opinion in Lipidology (13,1:41)

Eat, Drink, and Be Healthy, Simon & Schuster, New York, 2001

Effect of a Low Carbohydrate Ketogenic Diet Program on Fasting

Lipid Subfractions, Paper presented at: American Heart Association Scientific Sessions; November 17-20, 2002; Chicago

European Journal of Nutrition (40,6:289)

Journal of Natural Products (62,2:294)

Journal of Nutrition (132,5:1062S)

Journal of the American College of Nutrition (19,5:578)

Journal of the American Medical Association (280,23:2001)

Labeling and Marketing Information, The National Organic Program <www.ams.usda.gov/nop/FactSheets/LabelingE.html> retrieved Dec. 19, 2002

Michigan State University news release (Jan. 29, 1999)

Nutrition Reviews (60,6:170)

Penn State news release (Jan. 17, 2002)

Preventive Medicine (34,3:364)

Product Review: Garlic Supplements, ConsumerLab <www.consumerlab.com/results/garlic.asp> retrieved Oct. 30, 2002

Synergism Between Antiplatelet Properties of Grape Seed and Grape Skin Extracts, Paper presented at: Experimental Biology 2001; March 31-April 4, 2001; Orlando, Fla.

The New Pritikin Program, Pocket Books, New York, 1991

Breast cancer

American Institute for Cancer research news release (Sept. 12, 2002)

American Journal of Epidemiology (152,6:514)

Annals of Internal Medicine (137,10:798)

Appendix B. What Foods Are Good Sources of Vitamin A, Vitamin C, Calcium and Iron? Food and Nutrition Service – United States Department of Agriculture <www.fns.usda.gov/tn/Resources/appendb.pdf> retrieved Dec. 17, 2002

Asia Pacific Journal of Clinical Nutrition (11,1:79)

Cancer Epidemiology Biomarkers & Prevention (9,7:719; 11,5:451; 11,9:852)

Energy balance – an etiologic factor in human cancer: Randomized trial of exercise effect on breast cancer biomarkers, Paper presented at 18th UICC International Cancer Congress; July 3, 2002; Oslo, Norway

European Journal of Epidemiology (14,8:737)

FDA clears new device for radiation treatment for breast cancer, U.S. Food and Drug Administration <http://www.fda.gov/bbs/topics/ANSWERS/2002/ANS01150.html> retrieved Oct. 23, 2002

International Journal of Cancer (99,2:238)

Journal of Agricultural and Food Chemistry (50,23:6798)

Journal of Cellular Biochemistry (82,3:387)

Journal of the National Cancer Institute (94,17:1301)

More Color, More Health, National Center for Chronic Disease Prevention and Health Promotion <http://www.cdc.gov/nccdphp/dnpa/5ADay/campaign/color/greens.htm> retrieved Dec. 12, 2002

Nutrition Concepts and Controversies, Wadsworth/Thomson

Learning, Belmont, Calif., 2000

The Columbia University College of Physicians and Surgeons Complete Home Medical Guide, Crown Publishers, Inc., New York 1995

The National Academies news release (Sept. 5, 2002)

The Review of Natural Products, Facts and Comparisons, St. Louis, Mo., 2002

USDA Dietary Guidelines 2000 – Nutrition and Your Health, United States Department of Agriculture, Washington, DC 20250

United States Department of Agriculture Nutrient Data Laboratory <http://www.nal.usda.gov/fnic/foodcomp> retrieved Sept. 11, 2002

Wellness Foods A to Z, Rebus, Inc., New York, 2002

Cataracts

American Journal of Clinical Nutrition (75,3:540; 70,4:517)

Cataracts, American Academy of Ophthalmology, P.O. Box 7424, San Francisco, CA 94120

Citrus Fruits – citrus.spp, University of Georgia Department of Horticulture <http://www.uga.edu/fruit/citrus.htm> retrieved Oct. 30, 2002

Dietary Reference Intakes for Energy, Carbohydrate, Fiber, Fat, Fatty Acids, Cholesterol, Protein, and Amino Acids (Macronutrients) National Academies Press, Washington

Facts about vitamin A and carotenoids, NIH Office of Dietary Supplements <http://www.cc.nih.gov/ccc/supplements/vita.html> retrieved Feb. 15, 2001

Journal of Nutrition (132,6:1299)

Mango, Raw, USDA National Agricultural Library Food and Nutrition Information Center <http://www.nal.usda.gov/fnic/cgi-bin/list_nut.pl> retrieved Jan. 20, 2003

Maria Pastor-Valero, Senior Lecturer, Nutrition Department Faculty of Public Health University of São Paulo, São Paulo, Brazil

Mayo Clinic Guide to Self-Care, Mayo Foundation for Medical Education and Research, Rochester, Minn., 1999

The Complete Home Wellness Handbook, Rebus, Inc., New York, New York, 2001

United States Department of Agriculture Nutrient Data Laboratory <http://www.nal.usda.gov/fnic/foodcomp> retrieved Jan. 3, 2003

Colds and flu

Alternative Therapies in Health and Medicine (7,3:104)

American Family Physician (60,7:2061)

Andy Smith, Professor of Psychology, Cardiff University, Wales

Baker's Dozen Cold Remedies Still Work, Cedars-Sinai press release, Nov. 23, 1999

British Medical Journal (322,7298:1327)

Chest (118,4:1150)

Clinical Diagnostic and Laboratory Immunology (9,1:182)

European Journal of Clinical Nutrition (54,3:263)

Herbs of Choice, The Therapeutic Use of Phytomedicinals, The Haworth Press, Binghamton, N.Y., 1999

Influenza, Centers for Disease Control and Prevention, <www.cdc.gov/ncidod/diseases/flu/fluinfo.htm> retrieved Jan. 4, 2000

Journal of Alternative and Complementary Medicine (1,4:361)

Journal of the American Medical Association (288,12:1471)

Kansenshogaku Zasshi (71,6:487)

Medicine and Science in Sports and Exercise (30,11:1578)

Nutraceuticals, The Complete Encyclopedia of Supplements, Herbs, Vitamins, and Healing Foods, The Berkley Publishing Group, New York, 2001

Nutritional Neuroscience (5,2:145)

QJM (96,1:35)

The American Pharmaceutical Association, Practical Guide to Natural Medicines, William Morrow and Company, Inc., New York, 1999

The FASEB Journal Express Article (10.1096/fj.00-0721fje)

Colon cancer

Cancer Epidemiology, Biomarkers and Prevention (11,2:187; 11,3:227)

Estimation of the proportion of cancers preventable by dietary changes, Paper presented at: European Conference on Nutrition and Cancer; June 24, 2001; Lyon, France

Journal of Exposure Analysis and Environmental Epidemiology (11,3:155)

Nutrition and Cancer (40,2:125)

University of Texas Southwestern Medical Center news release (May 17, 2002)

What You Need to Know About Cancer of the Colon and Rectum, Publication No. 99-1552, National Cancer Institute, NCI Public Inquiries Office, Suite 3036A, 6116 Executive Boulevard, MSC8322, Bethesda, MD 20892-8322

Constipation

European Journal of Gastroenterology & Hepatology (14,9:991)

Depression

About ConsumerLab.com, ConsumerLab.com <www.consumer lab.com> retrieved Jan. 8, 2003

Alternative and Complementary Therapies (5,5:266)

Alternative Medicine Review (4,5:330)

Archives of General Psychiatry (59,10:913)

Bulletin of the Menninger Clinic (66,2:103)

Depression and Anxiety, The Johns Hopkins White Papers, MedLetter Associates, Inc., New York, 2001

Dietary Supplements, NSF International: The Public Health and Safety Company <www.nsfconsumer.org> retrieved Jan. 8, 2003

Duke University Medical Center news release (April 12, 2002)

Journal of the American Medical Association (287,14:1807)

National Institutes of Health news release (April 9, 2002)

Nutrition (16,7-8:544)

Nutrition Concepts and Controversies, Wadsworth/Thomson Learning, Belmont, Calif., 2000

PDR for Nutritional Supplements, Medical Economics Company, Inc., Montvale, N.J., 2001

Product Review: Omega-3 Fatty Acids (EPA and DHA) from Fish/ Marine Oils, ConsumerLab.com <www.consumerlab.com> retrieved Nov. 21, 2001

Product Review: SAM-e, ConsumerLab.com <www.consumer lab.com> retrieved March 30, 2000

S-Adenosyl-L-Methionine for Treatment of Depression, Osteoarthritis, and Liver Disease, Agency for Healthcare Research and Quality Publication No. 02-E034, U.S. Department of Health and Human Services, 2101 East Jefferson Street, Rockville, MD 20852

St. John's Wort and the Treatment of Depression, The National Center for Complementary and Alternative Medicine <http:// nccam.nih.gov> retrieved Jan. 9, 2003

The Annals of Pharmacotherapy (36,3:375)

The Complete German Commission E Monographs, American Botanical Council, Austin, Texas, 1998

Herbs of Choice, The Therapeutic Use of Phytomedicinals, The Haworth Press, Binghamton, N.Y., 1999

U.S. Pharmacopeia Dietary Supplement Verification Program, U.S. Pharmacopeia <www.usp.org> retrieved Jan. 8, 2003

Diabetes

Alternative Medicine Review (7,1:45)

American Chemical Society news release (May 20, 2002)

American Journal of Clinical Nutrition (76,1S:274S,290S)

Annals of the New York Academy of Science (967:329)

American Diabetes Association <www.diabetes.org> retrieved Jan. 27, 2003

Diabetes (51,6:1851)

Diabetes Care (25,1:148; 25,4:645)

European Journal of Human Genetics (10,11:682)

Harvard School of Public Health press release (Nov. 26, 2002)

Journal of the American Medical Association (288,20:2554)

Lancet (359,9309:824; 360,9344,1477)

Mount Sinai School of Medicine press release (Nov. 11, 2002)

Omega-3 PUFA Supplementation and Insulin Sensitivity, Paper presented at: Experimental Biology conference; Apr. 22, 2002; New Orleans

Proceedings of the National Academy of Science (99,24:15596)

University of Chicago news release (May 24, 2002)

University of Texas Southwestern Medical Center at Dallas news release (Feb. 5, 2002)

National Diabetes Information Clearinghouse <www.niddk.nih.gov> retrieved Nov. 5, 2002

Forgetfulness

Dr. Lon White, Pacific Health Research Institute, Honolulu

Journal of Ethnopharmacology (69,2:105)

Northumbria University press release (March 2002)

Annals of the New York Academy of Science (959:167)

Baycrest Center for Geriatric Care press release (Feb. 19, 2001)

Complementary Therapies in Medicine (8,1:2)

Neurobiology of Learning and Memory (75,2:179)

Psychological Science (12,6:516)

The Memory Bible, Hyperion, New York, 2002

University of Michigan news release (Oct. 22, 2002)

Gallstones

American Gastroenterological Association news release (Dec. 2, 2002)

Gastroenterology (123,6:1823)

International Journal of Cancer (102,4:407)

Joel Simon, M.D., Veterans Affairs Medical Center, San Francisco

University of California news release (Apr. 10, 2000)

Gout

American Journal of Physiology – Regulatory, Integrative and Comparative Physiology (283,5:R993)

Annals of the Rheumatic Diseases (59,7:539)

Arthritis, The Johns Hopkins White Papers, MedLetter Associates, Inc., New York, 2001

Current Opinions in Rheumatology (14,3:281)

Journal of Rheumatology (29,2:331)

Headache

Cleveland Clinic Journal of Medicine (68,11:904)

Headache (34,10:590; 41,9:899)

Journal of Ethnopharmacology (29,3:267)

Journal of Women's Health & Gender-Based Medicine (8,5:623)

Migraine Headaches, The National Women's Health Information Center <www.4woman.gov/faq/migraine.htm#5> retrieved Feb. 25, 2003

Neurology (50,2:466; 59,8:1289)

What You Should Know About Headache, The American Council for Headache Education <www.achenet.org/understanding> retrieved Feb. 24, 2003

Heartburn and Indigestion

American College of Gastroenterology news release (Oct. 21, 2002)

Archives of Surgery (136,9:1014)

Dr. Loren Laine, Professor of Medicine, Keck School of Medicine at the University of Southern California

Dr. Timothy C. Wang, Chief of the Division of Gastroenterology, University of Massachusetts Medical School

European Journal of Gastroenterology and Hepatology (14,9:991)

National Digestive Diseases Information Clearinghouse <www.niddk.nih.gov> retrieved Oct. 16, 2002

International Foundation for Functional Gastrointestinal Disorders news release (Nov. 19, 2001)

Nursing (31,6:46)

Scandinavian Journal of Gastroenterology (37,1:3)

Hiatal hernia

National Digestive Disease Information Clearinghouse <www.niddk.nih.gov> retrieved Dec. 10, 2002

Eat right – to stay healthy and enjoy life more, Arco Publishing, Inc., New York, 1979

The National Academies news release (Sept. 5, 2002)

High blood pressure

American Journal of Cardiology (65,10:45E)

American Journal of Hypertension (13,5Pt1:475)

Annals of Internal Medicine (131,1:21; 135,12:1019)

Annals of the New York Academy of Sciences (959:180)

Archives of Internal Medicine (160,6:837; 161,4:589; 161,5:685; 162,6:657; 162,19:2204)

British Medical Journal (323,7311:497)

Caffeine increases aortic stiffness in hypertensive patients, Paper presented at: Seventeenth Annual Scientific Meeting of the American Society of Hypertension; May 14-18, 2002; New York

Chronopharmacology of aspirin: administration-time dependent effects on blood pressure in women at high risk for preeclampsia, Paper presented at: Seventeenth Annual Scientific Meeting of the American Society of Hypertension; May 14-18, 2002; New York

Hypertension (38,6:1361)

Journal of Human Hypertension (7,1:33)

Journal of the American Medical Association (288,15:1882)

Magnesium: facts about dietary supplements, National Institutes of Health <www.cc.nih.gov/ccc/supplements/magn.html> retrieved Jan. 18, 2001

Medicine and Science in Sports and Exercise (33,11:1825)

Nature (419:685)

Pharmacological Research (41,5:555)

Use Seasonings Instead of Table Salt, American Heart Association <www.americanheart.org/presenter.jhtml?identifier=585> retrieved Jan. 23, 2002

Western Journal of Medicine (171,3:168)

High cholesterol

American Chemical Society news release (Nov. 7, 2001)

American Heart Association news release (March 22, 2002)

American Journal of Cardiology (70,15:1287; 86,12A:41L; 89,10:1201)

American Journal of Clinical Nutrition (53,5:1259; 71,5:1062; 72,5:1095; 74,5:596; 75,5:834; 76,2:326,351; 76,3:549)

American Journal of Medicine (112,5:343)

Atherosclerosis (161,2:395)

Avant Immunotherapies, Inc. press release (April 19, 1999)

British Medical Journal (323,7324:1286)

Circulation (102,18:2296; 106,11:1327)

Diabetes (51,8:2377)

Experimental Biology and Medicine (226,10:891)

Free Radical Research (35,6:967)

Journal of Agricultural and Food Chemistry (49,11:5315)

Journal of Clinical Endocrinology and Metabolism (87,4:1527)

Journal of Medicinal Food (5,1:1)

Journal of Nutrition (122,2:317; 131,9:2275,2358 and 132,4:703)

Journal of the American Dietetic Association (101,11:1319; 102,7:993)

Journal of the American Medical Association (275,6:447; 281,15:1387; 285,19:2486; 287,5:598)

Kansas State University news release (Oct. 25, 2001)

Life Sciences (62,24:PL381)

Lipids (37,3:245)

Oil, olive, salad or cooking, USDA Nutrient Database <www.nal.usda.gov/fnic/cgi-bin/nut_search.pl> retrieved Feb. 4, 2003

Postgraduate Medicine (112,2:13)

Preventive Medicine (28,4:333)

University of Illinois news release (April 8, 2002)

Insomnia

Annals of Internal Medicine (135,1:68)

Annals of the New York Academy of Sciences (957:341)

Appetite (37,3:249)

Applied Human Science (15,6:281)

Geriatrics (57,5:24)

Lippincotts Primary Care Practice (3,3:290)

Mayo Clinic news release (Feb. 14, 2002)

Primary Care (24,4:825)

Psychosomatic Medicine (64,3:407)

The Complete German Commission E Monographs, American Botanical Council, Austin, Texas, 1998

Tyler's Honest Herbal, The Haworth Herbal Press, New York, 1999

U.S. Pharmacist (26,6:50; 27,5:HS20)

Irritable bowel syndrome

Phytotherapy Research (15,1:58)

Kidney stones

American Journal of Kidney Diseases (40,2:265)

American Journal of Physiology, Regulatory, Integrative and Comparative Physiology (283,5R:993R)

Dr. Heinz Valtin, Professor Emeritus, Dartmouth Medical School

National Kidney and Urological Diseases Information Clear-inghouse <www.niddk.nih.gov> retrieved Jan. 7, 2003

USDA Nutrient Database for Standard Reference <www.nal.usda.gov/fnic/foodcomp> retrieved Jan. 10, 2003

Nutrition Concepts and Controversies, Wadsworth/Thomson Learning, Belmont, Calif., 2000

Nutrition Reviews (60,7:212)

The National Academies news release (Sept. 5, 2002)

University of Texas Southwestern Medical Center news release (Aug. 1, 2002)

Macular degeneration

Advances in Understanding Age-Related Macular Degeneration, Research to Prevent Blindness, 645 Madison Avenue, New York, NY 10022

American Journal of Clinical Nutrition (73:209)

Archives of Ophthalmology (119,10:1417)

British Journal of Ophthalmology (82,8:907)

Nutrition Concepts and Controversies, Wadsworth/Thomson Learning, Belmont, Calif., 2000

Nutritional reviews (60:283)

Ophthalmic and Physiological Optics (22,4:300)

Progress in Retinal and Eye Research (21:225)

U.S. Pharmacist (26,6:42)

Menopause

American Family Physician (66,1:129)

Annals of Internal Medicine (137,10:805)

Anticipated and unanticipated estrogenicity of several medicinal botanicals, Paper presented at American Association for Cancer Research annual meeting; April 6-10, 2002; San Francisco

Clover Isoflavones, Consumerlab.com <http://www.consumer-lab.com/results/phytoestrogens2.asp?> retrieved Aug. 16, 2001

Cynthia Ferrara, Assistant Professor, University of Maryland School of Medicine, Baltimore

Dietary Reference Intakes for Energy, Carbohydrate, Fiber, Fat, Fatty Acids, Cholesterol, Protein, and Amino Acids (Macronutrients), National Academies Press, Washington, 2002

FDA news release (Jan. 8, 2003)

Journal of Clinical Oncology (19,10:2739)

Journal of the American Medical Association (288,3:321; 288,3:334; 288,3:567)

Journal of Women's Health and Gender Based Medicine (11,2:163)

Maturitas (42,3:187)

Menopause (8,5:333)

Natural Woman, Natural Menopause, HarperCollins, New York, 1997

New England Journal of Medicine (345,1:34)

Pharmacopsychiatry (33,2:47-53)

The Columbia University College of Physicians and Surgeons Complete Home Medical Guide, Crown Publishers, Inc., New York, 1995

The Estrogen Decision, Westchester Publishing Company, Los Altos, Calif., 1994

The Review of Natural Products, Facts and Comparisons, St. Louis, Mo. 1998

USDA Dietary Guidelines 2000 – Nutrition and Your Health, United States Department of Agriculture, Washington, DC 20250

What Your Doctor May Not Tell You About Menopause, Warner Books, New York, 1996

Muscle cramps

Advances in Experimental Medicine and Biology (505:95)

American Society for Artificial Internal Organs Journal (38,3:M481)

European Journal of Clinical Nutrition (55,10:881)

Geriatrics (56,6:34)

Johns Hopkins Medical Institutions news release (Dec. 11, 2002)

USDA Nutrient Database for Standard Reference <www.nal.usda.gov/fnic/foodcomp> retrieved Feb. 24, 2003

Questions and Answers About Sprains and Strains, National Institute of Arthritis and Musculoskeletal and Skin Disease <www.niams.nih.gov> retrieved Nov. 14, 2002

University of Northern Iowa news release (Oct. 2, 2000)

Nausea and vomiting

About Nausea and Vomiting, The Cleveland Clinic <www.cleve
landclinic.org/health/health-info/docs/1800/1810.asp>
retrieved Jan. 21, 2003

American Family Physician (65,11:2307)

American Journal of Cardiology (90,3:248)

Bioscience (49,6:453)

Cornell University news release (March 4, 1998)

Dehydration Treatment Plans, Rehydration Project <www.rehy
drate.org/dehydration/treatment_plans.htm> retrieved Jan. 21,
2003

Dehydration, Medline Plus <www.nlm.nih.gov/medlineplus/
ency/article/000982.htm> retrieved Jan. 21, 2003

Journal of Nutrition (132,3:461)

Nausea and Vomiting, Medline Plus <www.nlm.nih.gov/medline
plus/ency/article/003117.htm> retrieved Jan. 21, 2003

New England Journal of Medicine (346,12:947)

Oral Rehydration Therapy, Net Scut <http://gucfm.george
town.edu/welchjj/netscut/fen/oral_rehydration.html>
retrieved Jan. 21, 2003

PDR for Herbal Medicines, Medical Economics Company,
Montvale, N.J., 1998

Psychiatry, W.B. Saunders Company, Philadelphia, 1997

Osteoarthritis

Alternative Medicine Review (4,5:330; 7,1:22)

Alternative Therapies in Health and Medicine (7,2:120,112)

American Journal of Physiology – Regulatory, Integrative and Comparative Physiology (283,5:R993)

Annals of Internal Medicine (133,8:635)

Archives of Physical Medicine and Rehabilitation (83,7:889)

Arthritis and Rheumatism (44,11:2531; 46,6:1544)

Arthritis Survival, Jeremy P. Tarcher/Putnam, New York, 2001

Arthritis, Consumer Health Information Research Institute <http://alhakelantan.tripod.com/healthremedies/id3.html> retrieved Jan. 15, 2003

Arthritis, The Johns Hopkins White Papers, MedLetter Associates, Inc., New York, 2001

Environmental Health Perspectives (102,S7:83S)

Inflammation Research (50,9:442)

Journal of Family Practice (51,5:425)

Journal of the American Osteopathic Association (102,5:283)

Lancet (357,9249:4)

Proceedings of the Society for Experimental Biology and Medicine (218,2:140)

Product Review: Glucosamine and Chondroitin, ConsumerLab.com <http://www.consumerlab.com/results/gluco.asp#tips> retrieved Jan. 15, 2003

Product Review: Omega-3 Fatty Acids (EPA and DHA) from Fish/ Marine oils, ConsumerLab.com <www.consumerlab.com/ results/omega3.asp?> retrieved Nov. 21, 2001

Ron Hobbs, Adjunct Basic Science Faculty, Bastyr University, Kenmore, Wash.

Nutrition Concepts and Controversies, Wadsworth/Thomson Learning, Belmont, Calif., 2000

The American Pharmaceutical Association's Practical Guide to Natural Medicines, William Morrow and Company, Inc., New York, 1999

Tyler Cymet, D.O., Associate Professor of Internal Medicine, Johns Hopkins School of Medicine, Baltimore

Herbs of Choice, The Therapeutic Use of Phytomedicinals, The Haworth Press, Binghamton, N.Y., 1999

U.S. Pharmacist (26,5:40)

Osteoporosis

American Journal of Clinical Nutrition (75,4:773; 76,1:187; 76,1:245; 76,6:1345)

American Journal of Epidemiology (155,7:636)

Archives of Internal Medicine (162,19:2217)

Archives of Physical Medicine and Rehabilitation (83,1:86)

Canadian Medical Association Journal (166,12:1517)

Chris Rosenbloom, Ph.D., R.D., Associate Dean, College of Health and Human Sciences and Associate Professor, Department of Nutrition, Georgia State University, Atlanta

Facts About Dietary Supplements: Vitamin D, National Institutes of Health <www.cc.nih.gov> retrieved Jan. 18, 2001

National Institutes of Health, Osteoporosis and Related Bone Diseases – National Resource Center <www.osteo.org> retrieved March 3, 2003

IFIC Review: Physical Activity, Nutrition and Bone Health, International Food Information Council Foundation <http://ific.org> retrieved April 3, 2002

Integrative Medicine Consult (4,7:84)

Journal of Clinical Endocrinology and Metabolism (87,5:2008)

Journal of Nutrition (132,11:3422)

Journal of the American College of Nutrition (21,2:97; 21,3:239; 21,5:388)

Medical Journal of Australia (177,3:139)

Medicine and Science in Sports and Exercise (34,1:17)

Osteoporosis: Progress and Promise, National Institute of Arthritis and Musculoskeletal and Skin Diseases, National Institutes of Health <www.niams.nih.gov> retrieved March 11, 2003

Proceedings of the National Academy of Sciences (99,21:13487)

South Dakota State University news release (Nov. 1, 2002)

Southern Medical Journal (93,1:2)

Terrence Diamond, Associate Professor of Endocrinology, University of New South Wales, Australia

The Columbia University College of Physicians and Surgeons Complete Home Medical Guide, Crown Publishers, Inc., New York, 1995

Tufts University news release (March 21, 2002)

University of California, San Francisco, news release (May 23, 2002)

USDA Nutrient Database for Standard Reference <www.nal.usda.gov/fnic/foodcomp> retrieved March 11, 2003

U.S. Pharmacist (26:9; 27:5)

Prostate cancer

Agricultural Research (49,9:22)

American Journal of Epidemiology (155,11:1023)

Curcumin (dihydroferuloyl-methane) enhances TRAIL-induced apoptosis in LNCaP human prostate cancer cells, Paper presented at the annual meeting of the American Association for Cancer Research; April 6-10, 2002; San Francisco

Fred Hutchinson Cancer Research Center news release (Aug. 6, 2002 and Jan. 4, 2000)

Journal of Agricultural and Food Chemistry (49,6:3051)

Journal of the National Cancer Institute (94,13:981)

Urology (58,5:723; 60,5:919)

Rheumatoid arthritis

Alternative Medicine Review (4,6:392)

Arthritis and Rheumatism (46,1:83)

Arthritis, The Johns Hopkins White Papers, MedLetter Associates, Inc., New York, 2001

David Trentham, Assistant Professor, Harvard University School of Medicine, Boston

Epidemiology (11,4:402)

Lancet Oncology (1:107)

Nutrition Concepts and Controversies, Wadsworth/Thomson Learning, Belmont, Calif., 2000

Ted Mikuls, M.D., MSPH, Assistant Professor of Medicine, University of Nebraska Medical Center, Omaha, Neb.

Sinusitis

American Journal of Epidemiology (150,11:1223)

American Journal of Respiratory and Critical Care Medicine (166,2:144)

Clinical Infectious Diseases (30,2:387)

Fact Sheet: Sinusitis, National Institute of Allergy and Infectious Diseases <www.niaid.nih.gov/factsheets/sinusitis.htm> retrieved Feb. 13, 2003

Health Watch: Featuring Winter Illness: Acute Sinusitis, Creighton University Student Health Services <www.creighton.edu/Stu dentHealthServices/HealthWatch/Winter/Sinusitis.html> retrieved Feb. 12, 2003

American Academy of Allergy, Asthma, and Immunology <www.aaaai.org> retrieved Feb. 18, 2003

RN (64,1:42)

The American Pharmaceutical Association Practical Guide to Natural Medicines, William Morrow and Company, Inc., New York, 1999

Skin cancer

Archives of Dermatology (136,8:989)

BMC Dermatology (1,3:electronic format)

British Medical Journal (324,7352:1526A)

Cancer Epidemiology, Biomarkers and Prevention (9,7:727)

Cancer Research (54,13:3428; 61,13:5002)

International Journal of Oncology (18,6:1307)

Journal of Chemical Education (77,10:1298)

Journal of Dermatological Science (23,Suppl1:S45)

Journal of Nutrition (131,5:1449)

Journal of the American Academy of Dermatology (44,3:425)

Journal of the American College of Nutrition (20,1:71)

Lancet (359,9316:1484)

Masamitsu Ichihashi, M.D., Ph.D., Professor, Division of Dermatology, Department of Clinical Molecular Medicine, Translational Medicine Faculty of Medicine, Kobe University School of Medicine, Kobe, Japan

Monash University news release (April, 2001)

More Color, More Health: Reds, Center for Disease Control <http://www.cdc.gov/nccdphp/dnpa/5ADay/campaign/color/reds.htm> retrieved Dec. 19, 2002

Mutation Research (422,1:191)

Nutrition and Cancer (32,2:71; 37,2:161)

Olive oil, Epicurious.com <http://food.epicurious.com/run/fooddictionary/browse?entry_id=9357> retrieved Jan. 17, 2003

Proceedings of the National Academy of Sciences (99,19:12455)

Skin Pharmacology and Applied Skin Physiology (14,6:358)

The Columbia University College of Physicians and Surgeons Complete Home Medical Guide, Crown Publishers, Inc., New York, 1995

The Complete Home Wellness Handbook, Rebus, Inc., New York, 2001

The Journal of Dermatology (27,11:691)

The New American Plate, American Institute for Cancer Research, 1759 R Street NW, P.O.Box 97167, Washington, DC 20090-7167

Wellness Foods A to Z, Rebus, Inc., New York, 2002

Mayo Clinic <www.mayoclinic.com> retrieved Oct. 18, 2002

Stroke

American Academy of Neurology news release (Aug. 12, 2002)

Archives of Neurology (57,10:1503)

Circulation (98,12:1198)

Emergency Medicine (33,1:29)

Environmental Nutrition (25,2:2)

Journal of Hypertension (18,4:411)

Journal of the American Medical Association (288,8:973)

Medicine and Science in Sports and Exercise (34,4:592)

Neurology (59,3:314)

New England Journal of Medicine (347,6:395)

Nutrition Reviews (59,1Pt1:24)

Proceedings of the National Academy of Sciences of the United States of America (99,13:9031)

Rowett Research Institute news release (July 10, 2000)

Stroke (31,10:2287; 33,2:513; 33,6:1568; 33,8:2086; 33,9:2165)

Stroke Risk Factors and Their Impact, National Stroke Association <www.stroke.org/stroke_risk.cfm> retrieved Feb. 19, 2003

Wasabi as functional food: An overview, Paper presented at: International Chemical Congress of Pacific Basin Societies; Dec. 14-19, 2000; Honolulu

Syndrome X

American Journal of Hypertension (15,9:780)

Diabetes Care (25,1:148; 25,9:1612)

Dr. Gerald Reaven, Professor Emeritus, Stanford University School of Medicine

Findings and Recommendations from the American College of Endocrinology Conference on the Insulin Resistance Syndrome, American Association of Clinical Endocrinologists <www.aace.com/pub/irscc/findings.php> retrieved Feb. 6, 2003

Insulin Resistance Syndrome, American Academy of Family Physicians <http://familydoctor.org/handouts/660.html> retrieved Feb. 5, 2003

Journal of the American Medical Association (287,16:2081)

Syndrome X: The Silent Killer, Simon & Schuster, Inc., New York, 2000

Ulcers

Archives of Internal Medicine (160,9:1349 and 162,11:1237)

Brazilian Journal of Medical and Biological Research (35,5:523)

European Journal of Gastroenterology and Hepatology (14,5:521)

Gut (50,1:61)

National Digestive Diseases Information Clearinghouse <www.niddk.nih.gov> retrieved Oct. 25, 2002

Hospital Practice (36,8:55)

Jed W. Fahey, plant physiologist, Johns Hopkins School of Medicine

Judith J. Petry, Medical Director, Vermont Healing Tools Project

Nutrition Concepts and Controversies, Wadsworth/Thomson Learning, Belmont, Calif., 2000

PDR for Herbal Medicines, Medical Economics Company, Montvale, N.J., 1998

Phytomedicine (8,1:16)

Proceedings of the National Academy of Sciences (99,11:7610)

The Review of Natural Products, Facts and Comparisons, St. Louis, Mo., 2002

University of Southern California news release (April 8, 2002)

USDA Nutrient Database for Standard Reference <www.nal.usda.gov/fnic/foodcomp> retrieved Dec. 18, 2002

Yale University news release (Oct. 30, 2001)

Urinary tract infections

Dr. Carole Gordon, Urologist, Waco, Texas

Emergency Medicine (34,5:33)

National Kidney and Urological Disease Information Clearing-house <www.niddk.nih.gov> retrieved Jan. 13, 2003

Interstitial Cystitis Association <www.ichelp.org> retrieved Jan. 13, 2003

Weight control

Aim for a Healthy Weight, National Heart, Lung, And Blood Institute <www.nhlbi.nih.gov> retrieved Dec. 18, 2002

Archives of Internal Medicine (160,14:2150; 161,17:2133; 161,9:1194)

British Journal of Psychiatry (176,1:72)

Calcium Checklist – Food Guide Pyramid, Virginia Cooperative Extension, Virginia State University, Petersburg, VA 23806

Cleveland Clinic Journal of Medicine (69,11:849)

Centers for Disease Control and Prevention <www.cdc.gov> retrieved Dec. 12, 2002

Eat More, Weigh Less: Dr. Dean Ornish's Life Choice Program for Losing Weight Safely While Eating Abundantly, HarperCollins Publishers, New York, 1993

International Journal of Obesity and Related Metabolic Disorders (24,12:1683; 26,3:384; 26,8:1129)

Journal of Clinical Endocrinology and Metabolism (85,12:4635)

Journal of Clinical Psychiatry (59,9:447; 61S,11:37)

Journal of Nutrition (130,2S:268S; 131,8:2078; 131,11:2848)

Journal of the American College of Nutrition (21,2:146S; 21,2:152S)

Journal of the American Dietetic Association (101,3:345; 101,9:1006; 102,5:645; 102,7:993)

Journal of the American Medical Association (287,18:2414; 288,4:1723)

Losing Weight: More Than Just Counting Calories, FDA Consumer, U.S. Food and Drug Administration <www.cfsan.fda.gov> retrieved Jan. 16, 2003

National Academies Institute of Medicine news release (Sept. 5, 2002)

Nutrition Concepts and Controversies, Wadsworth/Thomson Learning, Belmont, Calif., 2000

Nutrition Reviews (59,8{Pt.1}:247)

PDR Guide to Drug Interactions, Side Effects, Indications, Contraindications, Medical Economics Company, Inc., Montvale, N.J. 1997

Postgraduate Medicine (112,2:35)

The American Journal of Clinical Nutrition (51,6:1013; 74,2:197; 76,1:5; 76,1:290S; 76,3:659; 76,4:743)

The Food Lover's Companion, Epicurious <eat.epicurious.com> retrieved Jan. 17, 2003

The Glucose Revolution, The Authoritative Guide to the Glycemic Index, Marlowe and Company, New York, 1999

The New American Plate Brochure, The American Institute for Cancer Research, 1759 R Street NW, Washington, DC 20009

The Practical Guide: Identification, Evaluation, and Treatment of Overweight and Obesity in Adults, NIH Publication No. 00-4084, National Institutes of Health, National Heart, Lung, and Blood Institute, Bethesda, MD 20824-0105

National Heart, Lung, and Blood Institute <www.nhlbi.nih.gov> retrieved Nov. 8, 2002

Personality and Individual Differences Special Issue (31,3:361)

National Institute of Diabetes & Digestive & Kidney Diseases <www.niddk.nih.gov> retrieved Jan. 27, 2003

Ways to Win at Weight Loss, FDA Consumer, U.S. Food and Drug Administration <www.cfsan.fda.gov> retrieved Jan. 15, 2003

What is the Thyroid? The Thyroid Society for Education & Research <www.the-thyroid-society.org> retrieved Feb. 5, 2003

Index

A

Acetaminophen, high blood pressure and 151

Acid indigestion, *see* Heartburn and indigestion

Advanced glycation endproducts (AGEs), diabetes and 105-106

African plum tree, for prostate health 248

Age-related macular degeneration (AMD), *see* Macular degeneration

Alcohol
  Alzheimer's disease and 15
  breast cancer and 55-57
  cancer and 78
  cataracts and 65
  forgetfulness and 116
  gout and 126
  high blood pressure and 147, 153
  high cholesterol and 162
  insomnia and 173
  interstitial cystitis and 303
  irritable bowel syndrome and 177
  menopause and 195
  migraines and 130
  nausea and vomiting and 215
  osteoporosis and 229, 243
  Syndrome X and 289
  ulcers and 300

Allergies 1-9
  sinusitis and 261-262

Almonds
  for high cholesterol 157
  See also Nuts

Alzheimer's disease 11-17

Angelica root, for ulcers 295-296

Antioxidants
  for Alzheimer's disease 13
  for asthma 20-21
  for atherosclerosis 27
  for cancer 51-54, 77
  for cataracts 65-66
  for forgetfulness 109-110
  for high blood pressure 146
  for high cholesterol 159-161, 167
  for macular degeneration 187-190
  for osteoarthritis 219
  for rheumatoid arthritis 251-252, 254-256
  for skin cancer 266, 269-270
  for stomach cancer 298-299
  for stroke 279
  for ulcers 295-296
  for wrinkles 272-273

Anxiety, nausea and vomiting and 214

Apples
  for asthma 19-20
  for atherosclerosis 29
  for constipation 80
  for high cholesterol 157-158
  for prostate cancer 246

Arnica, for osteoarthritis 224

Arteriosclerosis, *see* Atherosclerosis

Arthritis, *see* Osteoarthritis, Rheumatoid arthritis, and Gout

Artichokes
  for heartburn and indigestion 138
  for irritable bowel syndrome 176

Artificial sweeteners
  interstitial cystitis and 303

D

E

F

G

N

Valerian *(continued)*
for menopause 199

Vision problems, *see* Cataracts and
Macular degeneration

Vitamin A
for asthma 21, 24
for cataracts 64
for diabetes 101
for macular degeneration 185
for ulcers 293
See also Beta carotene and
Carotenoids

Vitamin B12
deficiency and 294
for Alzheimer's disease 13
for depression 83-84
for osteoarthritis 222
for SAM-e absorption 90, 225
for stroke 279-280
See also B vitamins

Vitamin B2, *see* Riboflavin

Vitamin B3, *see* Niacin

Vitamin B6
for depression 83-84
for insomnia 170
for kidney stones 179-181
for stroke 279-280
See also B vitamins

Vitamin C
for allergies 8
for Alzheimer's disease 13
for asthma 20-21, 24
for atherosclerosis 33-34
for cancer 52
for cataracts 59-61
for colds and flu 70
for depression 85
for diabetes 103-104
for forgetfulness 109
for gallstones 117-118
for high blood pressure 146, 279
for iron absorption 85
for macular degeneration 187, 189
for muscle cramps 204-205
for osteoarthritis 219

for osteoporosis 238
for stomach cancer 299
for stroke 279
for urinary tract infections 301

Vitamin D
for calcium absorption 231
for menopause 197
for migraines 129
for osteoarthritis 219
for osteoporosis 231-233
for prostate cancer 249
for rheumatoid arthritis 256-257

Vitamin E
for Alzheimer's disease 12
for asthma 21, 24
for atherosclerosis 33
for cataracts 63-64
for diabetes 101
for forgetfulness 109
for high blood pressure 147
for high cholesterol 156, 160-161,
279·
for leg cramps 207
for macular degeneration 189
for menopause 197
for muscle cramps 203-204
for osteoarthritis 218, 222
for prostate cancer 247
for rheumatoid arthritis 252, 254
for stroke 276, 279

Vitamin K, for osteoporosis 235, 238

W

Walnuts
for high cholesterol 32, 156, 161
See also Nuts

Water
for atherosclerosis 35-37
for colds and flu 72
for colon cancer 78
for constipation 80
for gout 125

Z

Y